"Help Me Talk Right"

HOW TO CORRECT A CHILD'S LISP
IN 15 EASY LESSONS

by

Mirla G. Raz, M.Ed.

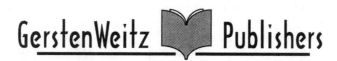
GerstenWeitz Publishers

P.O. Box 5599 • Scottsdale • Arizona • 85261-5599

Published by GerstenWeitz Publishing Company, P.O. Box 5599, Scottsdale, Arizona, 85261-5599.

Copyright * 1992 & 1993 by Mirla Geclewicz

Library of Congress Catalog Card Number: 92-63349

ISBN 0-9635426-0-5

Printed in the United States of America

Dear Reader,

"Will my child outgrow this speech problem?"

I cannot begin to count the number of times I have been asked this question. The reality is that some children do not outgrow their speech problems. It is critical that caring adults understand this and do whatever possible to help children with speech problems. No child today has to grow up with a lisp. Now anyone—clinic students, parents, speech pathologists, speech aides, teachers, teachers aides, and grandparents—can correct a child's lisp.

"Help Me Talk Right": How to Correct a Child's Lisp in 15 Easy Lessons is a speech correction program developed and used over the last 18 years in the public schools, at the UCLA Neuropsychiatric Institute, and in private practice. The simplicity of this program and the success of this approach have been the impetus for writing this book so that others may use it and help children. This program can be used for boys and girls who are four years old or older ("he" and "his" have been used generically in this book).

The "s" is the sound most frequently misarticulated by children. The lessons in this book will instruct you in how to correct a child's mispronounced "s" sound. They can also be used by parents of children receiving therapy from a speech pathologist. This book, used as a supplement, can enhance the progress of the child through speech therapy.

Try this book. I am sure you will derive tremendous satisfaction knowing you have helped a child correct a speech problem.

Sincerely yours,

Mirla G. Raz, M.Ed., CCC-SLP
Speech-Language Pathologist

ACKNOWLEDGEMENTS

I would like to express my deepest appreciation to the following people:

- My dedicated colleagues whose critical evaluations of the manuscript, input and suggestions improved the final product:
  Marilyn Lowell, MA, CCC-SP/A,
  Susan Wildman, MA, CCC-SP,
  Julie Budrzysky, MA, CCC-SP,
  Phyllis Benson, MA, CCC-SP, and
  Helen Sherman-Wade, MA, CCC-SP.
- My husband, Zohar, whose computer expertise and moral support have been invaluable.
- My daughters, Keren and Dannah, and my nieces, Lissy and Jessy Lane, whose pictures and writing adorn the cover.
- Chris Gakopoulos, my illustrator.

<u>CONTENTS</u>

Prelesson vii

Lesson 1 - Tongue and Teeth Positioning 1

Lesson 2 - Producing the SSSSS Sound 3

Lesson 3 - Initial SSSSS in Simple Syllables 7

Lesson 4 - Final SSSSS in Simple Syllables 11

Lesson 5 - Initial SSSSS in Simple Words......................... 15

Lesson 6 - Final SSSSS in Simple Words 19

Lesson 7 - Pairing Initial SSSSS Simple Words 23

Lesson 8 - Pairing Final SSSSS Simple Words 27

Lesson 9 - Medial SSSSS in Simple Words 31

Lesson 10 - Initial SSSSS in Simple Sentences 35

Lesson 11 - Final SSSSS in Simple Sentences 39

Lesson 12 - SSSSS Blends 43

Lesson 13 - Sentences Using Initial, Medial,
            and Final SSSSS and SSSSS in Blends 49

Lesson 14 - Using SSSSS While Playing 53

Lesson 15 - Using SSSSS in Conversation 57

Certificate of Achievement 63

Postlesson - Making Sure the Child Continues
            to Use the SSSSS Sound 65

Appendix A - Worksheets 67

Appendix B - Using SSSSS in Conversation 87

Appendix C - Activities & Materials 93

Appendix D - Lateral Lisp Supplement 95

PRELESSON

WHAT YOU NEED TO KNOW BEFORE BEGINNING THE LESSONS

The lessons you will soon begin will be easy to follow and understand after you have read the Prelesson. It is important that you read the entire Prelesson before beginning Lesson One.

IDENTIFYING A LISP

Most children who mispronounce the *s* sound protrude their tongue between their front teeth. When a child does this, his *s* sounds like a *th*. So, if the child is asked to say the word *some*, he will say *thumb*. A child who uses *th* in place of *s* is said to have a lisp. A child who lisps also protrudes his tongue on *z* so that the *z* sounds like *th* as in *that*.

Make sure the child you are working with has his front teeth. If the child is missing front teeth, wait until the child's front teeth have come in before attempting to determine whether the child lisps or before attempting to correct the lisp.

SSSSS AND ZZZZZ SOUNDS

So far, *s* and *z* have been used to indicate sounds when actually they are letters. As letters we call them *es* and *zee*. Because this book will focus on the <u>sounds</u>, sssss and zzzzz will be used instead of *s* and *z*. By placing your teeth together and forcing air out you will make the sssss sound just as you do when you say sssss in the word *sit*. Do the same and add voice (vibrate your vocal cords) and you will make the zzzzz sound just as you do when you say zzzzz in the word *zoo*. An easy way to understand the difference between the production of sssss and zzzzz is to place your palm lightly on your throat. Say sssss. You should not feel any vibration in your throat. Keep your palm on your throat. Say zzzzz. You should feel vibration. Sometimes a word is spelled with the letter *s* but the sound produced is zzzzz, as in *is* or *has*.
Note: In order to keep the text of the lessons simple, sssss will be written throughout this book but, in the process of doing the lessons, both sssss and zzzzz sounds will be corrected.

WHEN TO SEEK PROFESSIONAL HELP

A therapy program is started only after the problem has been identified. If you are certain the child you are working with lisps, you have identified the problem. There are, however, some children who lisp as well as incorrectly say other sounds. If a child has multiple speech errors, consult with a licensed speech pathologist (most, but not all, states license speech pathologists) or a certified speech pathologist before beginning this program. A speech pathologist certi-fied by the American-Speech-Language-Hearing Association will have the letters CCC following her name and degree (example: Mirla G. Raz, M.Ed., CCC). A speech pathologist will help you identify which sounds the child does not say correctly. She will also determine which sound should be corrected first. Once the speech pathologist recommends that the child's frontal lisp be corrected, feel free to begin Lesson One.

A speech pathologist should also be consulted if any of the following occurs as you do the lessons:

- You find that you and the child do not work well together, you are continually frustrated with the progress of the child, or the child is frustrated.
- You have been unable to accomplish the goal of a lesson after trying for about two weeks.

If you consult with a speech pathologist, tell her that you are working on a program to correct a child's lisp but that you and the child have reached an impasse. Ask the speech pathologist if you could set up an appointment for a consultation. When you meet with the speech pathologist, explain the problem. She may be able to help with the problem during the consultation or she may wish to work with the child for a session or two, until the problem you have presented is resolved. Once the speech pathologist has resolved the problem, you can continue with the next lesson in the book.

It is important that all children have their hearing checked to rule out a hearing loss which may be causing a speech problem. Many preschools and elementary schools offer routine hearing screenings, as do audiologists, speech pathologists in private practice, speech clinics, and pediatricians. A hearing screening will indicate only if the child may have a hearing loss. If the hearing screening indicates a possible hearing loss or if you suspect the child may have a hearing loss, then a complete audiological evaluation by a licensed or certified audiologist is recommended. An audiologist certified by the American Speech-Language-Hearing Association will have the letters CCC-A after her name and degree (example: Jane Smith, M.S., CCC-A).

WORKING WITH THE CHILD

It is important that anyone working with a child feel motivated to help the child. You must feel that what you are doing is valuable and will benefit the child. These feelings will be conveyed to the child through your words and attitude. If you feel motivated it will be much easier to motivate the child. If you consider the child's speech lessons to be important the child will take the cue from you. Once you have decided that you are ready to help the child, you need to tell him that you and he will work together so that he can learn to say his sssss sound the right way. Tell him that you and he will be playing games and looking at pictures and that the lessons will be fun.

Praise is an important motivator. Children who are motivated try to please the adult they are working with. Always remember that effort, as well as success, deserves praise. Tell the child frequently that he is doing a fine job. Avoid using the word "no." Instead say, "Try again," "Almost," or "Good try." Be positive and patient with the child. Impatience and/or a negative attitude will cause the child to resist doing the lessons and practice sessions.

Be alert and sensitive to the child. Motivation can wane if a child feels he is being challenged beyond his abilities. Children will get squirmy and begin to misbehave if they can no longer sit and concentrate or have lost interest. If a lesson time is 20 minutes and the child becomes squirmy after 10 minutes, take a break for a couple of minutes to "shake the squiggles out." The child will show you he has lost interest by not paying attention, fidgeting, or misbehaving. Once the child loses interest, it is best to end the session and resume the lesson later or the next day.

Maintain realistic expectations of what the child can do. After the first two or three lessons you may feel the urge to ask the child to repeat what he just told you, using his new sssss sound. For instance, the child wants to tell you about something that just happened. He lisps as he talks. You ask him to say it again but with his new sssss sound. *Avoid that temptation! Do not expect the child to use sssss in conversation because he has learned how to say sssss correctly.* Learning to use a new sssss sound is a process that is clearly laid out in this book. It may appear simple to you, as an adult, for the child to start using sssss in conversation now that he has learned how to make the sound. In reality, it is a giant leap to go from being able to say sssss to using it all the time when talking. An unrealistic expectation will only serve to frustrate you and the child. Besides, you will find that in no time the child will be ready for Lesson 15; this lesson makes using sssss in conversation fun for the child.

Do not attempt to correct any sound but the lisp while you are working on this program. Doing so will only serve to confuse and frustrate the child. Ignore any other speech errors he makes. Focus only on the sssss sound!

It is important to make each lesson fun. Fun is motivating. You can make each lesson fun by doing things the child enjoys. For instance, use board games if the child enjoys them. Have books and crayons available if the child enjoys coloring. More is said about suggested materials later on.

Enjoy playing and working with the child when you do the lessons, and have fun!

Let's review the important points to working with child:

- Feel motivated to help the child.
- Tell the child that you and he will be working on the sssss sound.
- Praise the child frequently.
- Be sensitive and alert to the child.
- Maintain realistic expectations.
- Make the lessons fun.

LESSONS

Lessons take anywhere from 10 to 30 minutes. Do not push the child past his limit. A session that is too long can frustrate the child and you. Try to do at least one, but no more than three, lessons each week. It is very important that you follow the lessons in order. Do not skip any. Correcting a child's lisp is a process which requires learning one task before the next can be added.

If you are a parent using this book, try to set aside the same time each day for a lesson or practice session. The child's speech sessions should be treated as ballet lessons, soccer practice, or any other scheduled activity, with its own special time during which NOTHING ELSE IS DONE. Do not push a lesson in when you or your child has a free moment or when you are, for instance, cooking or the child is taking a bath.

You and the child should not be distracted during the lessons and practice sessions. Make sure speech time with your child is free of common household distractions. Turn off the radio or television. Let the answering machine answer the phone for you, if you have one. If you must answer the phone tell your caller that you cannot talk and you will call back. If there are other children at home make sure they are occupied during the lesson and practice session times. Older children can read or play in another room of the house. It may be best to do a lesson or practice session during a younger sibling's nap time.

Lessons should be done at a table, preferably a child's table. Make sure the child sits comfortably and is high enough to easily see any game, toy, and/ or worksheet that is on the table before him.

Each lesson states the goal of the lesson, the materials you will need, and how long the lesson will take. The instructions for each lesson, after Lesson 1, are broken down into steps.

Step One, for most lessons, will ask you to review a previous lesson or lessons. You should review the previous lesson by asking the child to do a few items of that lesson. For instance, one row of the worksheet can be done. *You do not need to do the entire worksheet when you review.*

If the child has difficulty with a lesson you will find help in **Troubleshooting.** Lessons Two through Fourteen have Troubleshooting sections you can refer to; they can be found after the Practice Sessions. *The Troubleshooting section will instruct you how to make the lesson easier for the child.* Refer to the Troubleshooting section if after a few attempts the child is unable to perform the task correctly. Each lesson tells you when to refer to Troubleshooting for that lesson.

Students in Clinic

Students in clinic may find that their scheduled appointment with the child runs longer than the lesson time needed to complete a lesson. In other words, the child is scheduled for an hour of clinic therapy but the lesson is only 10 minutes long. If the child is receiving speech therapy only for a lisp and in the student's judgment the child is capable of moving on, the student may attempt to move on to the next lesson. If you, the student, decide to do more than one lesson during a therapy session, be certain that the child has met the goal of the lesson just completed before you move him on. Remember to be sensitive to the child. You want to challenge him without frustrating him. Stop and go back to the previous lesson if the child indicates, through his responses and behavior, that he is not ready for the next lesson. Instruct the parents to do the Practice Sessions for the last lesson successfully completed.

MATERIALS

Each lesson will tell you which category of materials, turn-taking activities, or conversational activities to use. Activities and toys are used to make the lessons fun for the child. Prepare the materials you will be using for the Lesson before you sit down with the child. Below are examples of different activities and toys. Feel free to be innovative. Better yet, let the child decide which activity or toy he wishes to use. See Appendix C for additional ideas.

Turn-taking Activities: You will need turn-taking activities for Lessons 2 through 12. These materials should be appropriate for the child's age and easy for the child to follow, and should allow the child and you to take turns at play. Taking a turn should be used as a reward for success. For example, the child said sssss in isolation five times, as you asked him to do. He can take a turn. Then you take a turn. Taking a turn should also be a reward for effort even if the goal has not been met. Try to finish the lesson and the turn-taking activity at the same time. As you do the lessons there will be reminders to take turns at the turn-taking activity. Some examples of turn-taking materials are:

- Board games (Candyland, Chutes and Ladders, Pizza Party, checkers, etc.)
- Coloring book and crayons (The child colors in only a segment of the picture each turn.)
- Memory Game
- Legos, blocks, logs, etc. (The child adds a few pieces at each turn to what he is building.)
- Puzzles

Conversational Activities: These are not turn-taking activities. Instead, these materials and activities are used to stimulate the child to talk. You will use them for Lesson 14. Some examples of conversational materials and activities are:

Playing with dolls or action figures	Playing school
Talking about pictures	Reading a book together
Playing house	Playing with cars

PRACTICE SESSIONS

Practice sessions are important for reinforcement and carryover of each lesson.
A successful lesson must be practiced a few times before the next lesson is attempted. If the child completes a lesson on Monday, he should practice what he has learned on Tuesday and Wednesday. A practice session is handled like a lesson except that nothing new is learned. Each lesson will tell you about the practice sessions for that lesson.

Do one practice session a day. The first practice session should be done the day after the lesson. For example, if the child does Lesson 5 on Monday, the first practice session should be done on Tuesday, the second practice session on Wednesday, and so on. The next lesson can be taught after the practice sessions have been completed.

If you are not the parent, instruct the parent to do the practice sessions at home. The practice sessions are important for reinforcement and carryover. Explain to the parent what you would like done. It is important that you also show the parent how you would like the practice session done. If the lesson calls for a turn-taking activity, ask the parent to use one as well and instruct her how to incorporate it into the practice session. Show the parent how to use the worksheet. If the lesson calls for reinforcers, explain to the parent what reinforcers are and how to use them. I always request that the parent bring a notebook to speech. I then write in the notebook what I would like the parent to do at home with the child. Using a notebook also allows me to easily and quickly refer to what I had asked the parent to do.

Allow the parent, when a worksheet is needed, to take the applicable worksheet(s) home until the child's next speech session.

WORKSHEETS

There are nine worksheets. They can found at the back of the book in Appendix A. You will need a worksheet for most lessons. Each lesson will tell you which worksheet you will need for that lesson. Copy or cut out the worksheet you will need, and place it in front of the child before you begin the lesson. **Save each worksheet.** You will be using many of them for lessons farther on in the book.

If you are a student, you might want to laminate the worksheets. This will protect them and allow you to reuse them. Laminating will also make the worksheets easy to wipe clean of crayon and other marks.

PRAISE, REWARDS, AND REINFORCERS

Praise is extremely important. The child will know he is successful when he is praised. Because praise is so important, there will be frequent reminders, in each lesson, to praise the child. Praise comes in many forms. It can be verbal as when you say, "Great work!" or "What a good sssss!" Parents can use hugs and kisses accompanied by verbal praise.

- Be generous with praise.
- Avoid showing frustration, yelling, or punishing the child if he is having difficulty with a lesson. Patience will pay off.

Rewards and reinforcers will be explained in the applicable lessons.

CHECKLISTS

The Prelesson Checklist, below, goes over important points discussed in the Prelesson. The Progress Checklist, on the following page, will help you keep track of the lessons completed. Feel free to remove it and keep it in a handy place if that is more convenient for you than leaving it in the book.

PRELESSON CHECKLIST

Place a check on each line.

_____I have explained to the child that I will help him learn to say sssss correctly.

_____I will be patient and sensitive as I work with the child.

_____I know what to do when the child is no longer interested in continuing the session.

_____I will set aside a specific time of day, each day, to work on the lessons and practice sessions.

_____I will use praise often as I work with the child.

_____I will make the lessons and practice sessions fun.

LET'S START LESSON 1!

PROGRESS CHECKLIST

(Use this checklist to keep track of the chilld's progress.)

Lesson	Completed (✔)	Practice Session (cross out as completed)	
1		1 2	Good job. You are ready for the next lesson.
2		1 2	Move on to Lesson 3.
3		1 2	Good work! Moving right along.
4		1 2 3	Ready for words.
5		1 2 3	Nice work!
6		1 2 3	Let's pair in the next lesson.
7		1 2 3	Keep up the good work.
8		1 2	More than halfway through!
9		1 2	Sentences next. No problem.
10		1 2	Great job!
11		1 2	Getting close to the end.
12		1 2 3	The final stretch.
13		1 2 3	The next to last lesson is next.
14		1 2 3 4 5	The light at the end of the tunnel.
15		60 pennies 10 nickels	Congratulations! You did it!

TONGUE AND TEETH POSITIONING

1

GOAL

You will teach the child to keep his teeth together and his tongue behind his teeth.

MATERIALS

Mirror
Worksheet 1
Marker or crayon

LESSON TIME

10 minutes

WHAT TO DO

Sit next to the child. Place the mirror in front of you and the child. Look in the mirror, with the child, and say:
"Look at my teeth. I'm going to make believe my teeth are a cage. I'm going to make believe my tongue is a tiger.

"When I open the cage (open teeth) you can see the tiger (wiggle tongue). When the cage is open the tiger can come out (stick out tongue). Before I close the cage I let the tiger lie down (place tongue at the bottom of mouth behind lower front teeth). Then I close the cage (place tongue at bottom of mouth and shut teeth with upper teeth overlapping lower teeth). When the cage is closed the tiger cannot come out (place tongue again at bottom of mouth and shut teeth).

"Watch my mouth again. When I open the cage (open teeth slightly) the tiger comes out (protrude tongue). When my teeth are closed the tiger cannot come out (place tongue at bottom of mouth and shut teeth).

"Now it's your turn. Show me how you open your cage. Good job. Now show me how the tiger can come out of the cage. Good. Now lay the tiger down. Now shut the cage. Can the tiger come out? No. Let's try opening the cage again but this time only a little bit. Show me how the tiger can come out. Very good. Now lay the tiger down and shut the cage. Can the tiger come out? No.

"Show me again what the cage looks like when it is closed. Now show me what happens when the cage opens a little. Does the tiger come out? Yes. Let's practice laying the tiger down and closing the cage five times. Every time you lay the tiger down and close the cage, so that the tiger cannot come out, we will color a happy face in one of the circles," (Worksheet 1).

day until you feel the child is ready to move on to

PRODUCING THE SSSSS SOUND

GOAL

You will teach the child how to make the sssss sound.

MATERIALS

Turn-taking activity
Mirror

LESSON TIME

15 minutes

WHAT TO DO

Step One

Place the mirror in front of you and the child. Tell the child to <u>listen carefully and watch you. Place your teeth together and make an sssss sound. Repeat a few times.</u>
Tell the child that you could make that sound because the tiger was lying down, the cage was closed and the tiger did not come out.

⇩   ⇩   ⇩   ⇩   ⇩

Step Two

Ask the child to look in the mirror. Then ask him to make the sssss sound with you and to make his sssss so it sounds just like yours. Together make the sssss sound a few times. Allow the child to take a turn at the activity he selected. Then you take a turn. If the child makes a sound more like *sh* (as in "show") or is unclear, see Troubleshooting. If his sssss sounds good, continue to Step Three.

⇩   ⇩   ⇩   ⇩   ⇩

Step Three

Ask the child to make the sssss sound alone. If he is successful, ask him to make 5 sssss sounds in a row. Take turns at the activity. Continue this step until either the game is over or the child has lost interest.

If on his own the child protrudes his tongue, return to making the sound together. Take turns at the turn-taking activity. Repeat this step as often as necessary until the child is able to produce sssss on his own.

The child will need to practice producing sssss over the next two days before you move on to the next lesson. The idea is to carry over and reinforce correct production of the sssss sound.

Practice Session 1 is done the day after the lesson. Practice Session 2 is done the day after Practice Session 1. As much time should be spent on the Practice Sessions as was spent on the lesson.

If you are not the parent, it is important that you instruct the parent. Tell the parent what you would like done and how to do each practice session.

👍 👌 👍 👌 👍

Repeat the lesson once in the morning and once in the afternoon.

**Practice
Session 1**

👍 👌 👍 👌 👍

You will need about 10 pennies.

**Practice
Session 2**

Face the child so that he can see your mouth. Tell the child that you and he are going to play the "Catch Me" game. Tell him that you will try to trick him and he has to catch you. Tell the child that each time he catches you he will win a penny.

Tell the child that sometimes you will say sssss the right way with your teeth together (demonstrate). When you say sssss the right way, he should say, "Good talking." If he catches you saying sssss the right way, he will win a penny. Then tell him that sometimes you will say sssss the wrong way. Tell the child that instead of sssss you will say *th* (demonstrate). When you say *th*, he has to catch you. When he catches you he says, "Wrong." Tell the child that he will win a penny when he catches you saying sssss the wrong way. When he catches you saying *th*, ask him to help you say it correctly. Then say sssss together. Do a couple of practice trials with the child, using pennies, so that you are sure he understands what he has to do when you say sssss and *th*. Switch roles after the child has caught you a few times. This time the child tries to trick you. The child will enjoy giving you pennies for catching him say sssss correctly and incorrectly. Play "Catch Me" for about 10 minutes.

TROUBLESHOOTING

Some children do not make a clear sssss sound because their tongue is not in the correct position. You can help the child place his tongue in the correct position by doing the following:

1. Place a small dab of peanut butter behind the child's lower front teeth.
2. Ask the child to touch the peanut butter with his tongue. The child's tongue should now be at the bottom of his mouth. Using the mirror, show the child where his tongue should be when he shuts his teeth.
3. Ask the child to shut his teeth. Remind him to keep his tongue down while touching the peanut butter spot when he says sssss.
4. Ask the child to "make a big smile" (demonstrate by smiling broadly with the child) and make the sssss sound with you.

Repeat numbers 1-4 above a few times. When you feel your child is ready, do only numbers 3 and 4 above. If he is succeeds in making a clear sssss without the peanut butter, return to Step Two of the lesson. If his sssss still sounds like a *sh* or is not yet clear, continue to do numbers 1-4 until he is able to produce a clear sssss without the peanut butter. Then return to Step Two of the lesson.

Do not ask or expect the child to use sssss in conversation yet.

INITIAL SSSSS IN SIMPLE SYLLABLES

GOAL

You will teach the child to use initial sssss in combination with a vowel. (The sssss sound will be followed by a vowel sound.)

MATERIALS

Mirror
Turn-taking Activity

LESSON TIME

15 to 20 minutes

WHAT TO DO

Step One   Look in the mirror with the child. Ask the child to say his sssss sound the new way. If he is able to make the sssss sound five times, continue to Step Two. If he is unable to say the sssss sound five times, review Lesson 2 until he is able to say the sssss sound five times. **Do not move on to Step Two until the child is able to say sssss five times in a row.**

⇩   ⇩   ⇩   ⇩   ⇩

Step Two   You will now help the child learn to use sssss in combination with different vowel sounds. The child will be combining sssss with:

a as in "ape." This *a* will be shown as ā.
e as in "eat." This *e* will be shown as ē.
i as in "ice." This *i* will be shown as ī.
o as in "old." This *o* will be shown as ō.
o as in "shoe." This *o* will be shown as o͞o.

Look in the mirror with the child. Ask the child to repeat each sssss + vowel after you: *sā, sē, sī, sō, so͞o.* If the child correctly says the sssss with each vowel, praise him and allow him to take a turn at the turn-taking activity. Repeat this step until the turn-taking activity is completed or the child has indicated he is no longer interested in continuing. See Troubleshooting if the child lisps when producing these syllables.

PRACTICE SESSIONS 1 AND 2

The child may select a turn-taking activity if he wishes. Ask him to repeat each sssss + vowel combination after you, just as was done for the lesson. Praise the child for a job well done. If you are playing a game, allow him to take a turn at the game after he has repeated two or three sssss + vowel combinations.

TROUBLESHOOTING

Some children have difficulty making the transition from the sssss to the next sound. You can make this easier for the child by inserting a pause between the sssss and the vowel which follows.

Ask the child to say the sssss sound, then the ā sound. Demonstrate this step by doing the following: Say the sssss sound, pause, then say ā. Ask the child to do the same. Praise him for a successful attempt.

You will now ask the child to combine the sssss sound with the other vowel sounds. You will say each sssss sound, pause, then say one of the vowel sounds. The child will repeat what you have just said in the way you presented it. Continue until you have combined, and the child has repeated, each sssss + vowel combination. Remember to praise the child. He can take a turn at the activity each time he repeats, after you, an sssss + vowel series. As this step becomes easier for the child, decrease the pause time between the sssss sound and the vowel. Your child will be ready to return to Step Two once he can say: sā, sē, sī, sō, sōō.

Do not ask or expect the child to use sssss in conversation yet.

FINAL SSSSS IN SIMPLE SYLLABLES

 GOAL

You will teach the child to use final sssss in combination with a vowel. (The sssss sound will follow the vowel sound.)

 MATERIALS

Mirror
Turn-taking Activity

 LESSON TIME

15 to 20 minutes

WHAT TO DO

Step One   Review all the initial sssss simple syllables learned in Lesson Three. Praise the child for a job well done and allow him to take a turn at the activity selected. Move on to Step Two. If the child has difficulty using initial sssss in simple syllables, continue to review Lesson Three. *You may, however, continue to Step Two below.*

⇩   ⇩   ⇩   ⇩   ⇩

Step Two   You will now help the child learn to use final sssss in combination with different vowel sounds. The child will be combining sssss with:

   a as in "ape." This *a* will be shown as ā.
   e as in "eat." This *e* will be shown as ē.
   i as in "ice." This *i* will be shown as ī.
   o as in "old." This *o* will be shown as ō.
   o as in "shoe." This *o* will be shown as o͞o.

Look in the mirror with the child. Ask the child to repeat each vowel + sssss after you: ās, ēs, īs, ōs, o͞os. If the child correctly says the sssss with each vowel, praise him and allow him to take a turn at the turn-taking activity. Repeat this step until the activity is completed or the child has indicated he is no longer interested in continuing. If the child lisps when producing these syllables, see Troubleshooting.

PRACTICE SESSIONS 1 AND 2

The child may select a turn-taking activity if he wishes. Ask the child to repeat the vowel + sssss combinations after you, just as you did for the lesson. Praise him for a job well done. If a turn-taking activity was selected, allow him to take a turn at the turn-taking activity.

TROUBLESHOOTING:

Some children have difficulty making the transition from any sound to the sssss sound. You can make this easier for the child by inserting a pause between the vowel sound and the sssss.

Ask the child to say the $\bar{a}$, then sssss. Demonstrate this by doing the following: Say the $\bar{a}$, pause, then say sssss. Ask the child to do the same. Praise for a successful attempt and allow the child to take a turn.

You will now ask the child to combine the other vowels with sssss. You will say a vowel sound, pause, then sssss. The child will repeat what you have just said and the way you presented it. Continue until you have combined, and the child has repeated, each vowel + sssss combination. Remember to praise the child. He can take a turn at the activity each time he repeats a vowel + sssss series. As this step becomes easier for the child, decrease the pause time between the vowel and the sssss. Your child will be ready to return to Step Two once he can say $\bar{a}$s, $\bar{e}$s, $\bar{\imath}$s, $\bar{o}$s, $\overline{oo}$s without the pause.

Do not ask or expect the child to use sssss in conversation yet.

INITIAL SSSS IN SIMPLE WORDS

5

GOAL

You will teach the child how to say initial sssss in simple words.

MATERIALS

Turn-taking Activity
Worksheet 2

LESSON TIME

Approximately 20 minutes

WHAT TO DO

Step One   Review initial and final sssss in simple syllables in Lessons 3 and 4. Praise the child for a job well done. Allow him to take a turn at the activity selected. Move on to Step Two. **If the child has difficulty using initial sssss in simple syllables, return to Lesson 3. Do not continue with Lesson 5 until the child successfully completes Lesson 3.**

If the child has difficulties with <u>final</u> sssss in simple syllables, continue to work on Lesson 4. *You may, however, continue to Step Two.*

⇩   ⇩   ⇩   ⇩   ⇩

Step Two   You will now help the child use initial sssss in simple words. Place Worksheet 2 in front of the child. Worksheet 2 is made up of pictures whose names begin with the sssss sound. Tell the child that he will now need to remember to use sssss in words. Tell him that all the pictures on the worksheet begin with the sssss sound. You name the first picture. The child names the picture after you. If he has named the picture using a correct sssss, praise him. Do the next two pictures. Allow the child to take a turn at the turn-taking activity after he has named three pictures. You also take a turn. You continue in this way until you and the child have named each picture. Remember to take turns at the selected activity.

Review the sheet a second time, taking turns at the selected activity.

Go over the sheet a third time, but this time you point to each picture and the child tries to name it on his own. If he has difficulty with a picture you name it and he will name it after you.

See Troubleshooting if the child lisps when repeating each word or has difficulty repeating sssss in simple words.

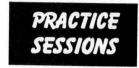

Reminder: Practice Session 1 is done the day after the Lesson, Practice Session 2 the day after Practice Session 1 and Practice Session 3 the day after Practice Session 2. Practice Sessions should last about 20 minutes each.

Practice Session 1

Look through magazines, newspapers, catalogues, etc., with the child. Look for 10 pictures that begin with sssss followed by a vowel (a, e, i, o, u). <u>DO NOT</u> select pictures that begin with *str* as in "straw," *spr* as in "spring," *scr* as in "scratch," *st* as in "step," *sp* as in "spill," *sk* as in "skate," *sw* as in "sweat," *sn* as in "snow," *sm* as in "small," *sl* as in "sleep," or *sh* as in "sheet."

As you and the child find initial sssss pictures, do the following:
1. You name the picture.
2. The child names the picture.
3. The child cuts and pastes the picture on a piece of paper. (Some children may need adult assistance with cutting and pasting.)
4. The child names each picture, using a correct sssss, that he has pasted.

Practice Sessions 2 & 3

Use Worksheet 2 and the pasted pictures. Place Worksheet 2 and pasted pictures in front of the child. Point to any initial sssss picture and ask the child to name it. Continue pointing, with the child naming, until the child has completed naming the pasted pictures and the pictures on Worksheet 2 or he indicates he has lost interest. A variation of the above is asking the child to point to and name any three pictures he wishes. Continue in this way until the activity is completed or the child indicates that he has lost interest.

TROUBLESHOOTING

Some children have difficulty connecting the sssss into a word. The child is accustomed to naming words with his old sound, and to say the word a different way may be confusing. You can help the child get over this difficulty by using a pause, as you did in Lessons 3 and 4. As you say each word, separate the sssss from the rest of the word. In other words, say sssss, wait 2 seconds and say "un" for "sun." The child repeats the word with the pause. Below are examples for a few more words:

sssss	(2-second pause)	"and" for "sand"
sssss	(2-second pause)	"ock" for "sock"
sssss	(2-second pause)	"oap" for "soap"

Continue in this way for all the pictures. Gradually reduce the pause until the child can name each picture without a pause. Once this occurs, return to Step One. Do not be concerned if the child needs to stay in Troubleshooting a few days. He can still do the Practice Sessions using the pause and later without the pause.

Do not ask or expect the child to use sssss in conversation yet.

FINAL SSSSS IN SIMPLE WORDS

 ☆ **GOAL**

You will teach the child how to say the final sssss sound in simple words.

  MATERIALS

Turn-taking Activity
Worksheet 3

 LESSON TIME

Approximately 20 minutes

WHAT TO DO

Step One   Review final sssss in simple syllables in Lesson 4 and initial sssss in simple words in Lesson 5. Praise the child for a job well done. Allow him to take a turn at the activity selected. Move on to Step Two. If the child has difficulty using <u>final</u> sssss in simple syllables, return to Lesson 4. **Do not move on to Step Two until the child is successful at Lesson 4.**

If the child has difficulty using <u>initial</u> sssss in simple words, continue to do Lesson 5. *You may, however, continue to Step Two if the child succeeded in completing Lesson 4.*

⇩   ⇩   ⇩   ⇩   ⇩

Step Two   You will now help the child use final sssss in simple words. Place Worksheet 3 in front of the child. Worksheet 3 is made up of pictures whose names end with the sssss sound. (Note: The sssss sound is the last sound, not necessarily the last letter. Many of the words end in the letter "e," which is silent.)

You name the first picture. The child names the picture after you. Allow the child to take a turn at the turn-taking activity after he has named three pictures. You also take a turn. Continue in this way until you and the child have named each picture. Remember to take turns at the selected activity. Review the sheet a second time, taking turns at the selected activity. Go over the sheet a third time, but this time you point to each picture and the child tries to name it on his own. If he has difficulty with a picture, you name it and ask him to name it after you.

See Troubleshooting if the child lisps when repeating each word or has difficulty repeating final sssss in simple words.

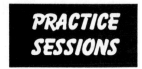

Look through magazines, newspapers, catalogues, etc., with the child. Look for 10 pictures which end in the sssss sound.

Practice Session 1

As you and the child find final sssss pictures, do the following:
1. You name the picture.
2. The child names the picture.
3. The child cuts and pastes the picture on a piece of paper. (Some children may need adult assistance with cutting and pasting.)
4. The child names each picture, using a correct sssss, that he pasted.

Praise the child for a job well done.

Use Worksheet 3 and the pasted pictures. Place the worksheet and pasted pictures in front of the child. Point to a final sssss picture and ask the child to name it. Continue pointing, as the child names pictures, until the child has completed naming the pasted pictures and the pictures on Worksheet 3 or the child indicates he has lost interest. Praise the child for a job well done. A variation of the above is asking the child to point to and name any three pictures he wishes. Continue in this way until the activity is completed or the child indicates that he has lost interest.

Practice Sessions 2 & 3

TROUBLESHOOTING

Some children have difficulty connecting the sssss into a word. The child is accustomed to naming words with his old sound, and to say the word a different way may be confusing. You can help the child get over this difficulty by using a pause, as you did in Lessons 3, 4, and 5. Use Worksheet 3. As you say each word, separate the sssss from the rest of the word. In other words, say the word without the sssss at the end, wait two seconds, then say sssss. For example, for the word "bus," say bu, wait two seconds, then say sssss. Your child repeats the word with the pause. Below are examples for a few more words:

hou	(2-second pause)	sssss for "house"
ga	(2-second pause)	sssss for "gas"
goo	(2-second pause)	sssss for "goose"

Continue in this way for all the pictures on the worksheet. Gradually reduce the pause until the child can name each picture without a pause. Once this occurs, return to Step One. Do not be concerned if the child needs to stay in Troubleshooting a few days. He can still do the Practice Sessions using the pause and later without the pause.

Do not ask or expect the child to use sssss in conversation yet.

PAIRING INITIAL SSSSS SIMPLE WORDS

 GOAL

You will teach the child how to combine two words that begin with the sssss sound.

 MATERIALS

Turn-taking Activity
Worksheet 2

 LESSON TIME

Approximately 20 minutes

WHAT TO DO

Step One   Review initial and final sssss in simple words in Lessons 5 and 6. Praise the child for a job well done. Allow him to take a turn at the activity selected. Move on to Step Two. If the child has difficulty using <u>initial</u> sssss in simple words, return to Lesson 5. **Do not move on to Step Two until your child is successful at Lesson 5.**

If the child has difficulty using <u>final</u> sssss in simple words, continue to do Lesson 6 until the child is successful. *You may, however, also move on to Step Two if the child succeeded in completing Lesson 5.*

⇩   ⇩   ⇩   ⇩   ⇩

Step Two   You will now help the child pair initial sssss simple words. Place Worksheet 2 in front of the child. Each picture on the sheet will be paired with one of the following initial sssss words: **see, say, sew, sit.** As you point to the pictures in each row you will say:

First Row:	*see sand, see sock, see soap, see sun*
Second Row:	*say seal, say saw, say seven, say soup*
Third Row:	*sew safe, sew sail, sew suit, sew sofa*
Fourth Row:	*sit sink, sit salt, sit saddle, sit soda*

Begin with the first row. Point to the first picture. Say the paired words. Ask the child to say what you said. Make sure he uses initial sssss in both words of the pair. You and the child take turns at the turn-taking activity. Continue if the child pairs without difficulty. See Troubleshooting if the child has difficulty saying sssss in both words.

⇩   ⇩   ⇩   ⇩   ⇩

Step Three   Now point to each picture and say the word pairs for each picture in the rest of the row. The child will repeat the word pair for each picture after you. Take turns at the turn-taking activity after you complete the row.

Move on to the second row of pictures. Point and say the word pair for each picture. The child will repeat the word pair for each picture after you. Take turns at the turn-taking activity after you complete the row. Do rows 3 and 4 as you did rows 1 and 2. Remember to praise the child for a job well done.

PRACTICE SESSIONS

Practice the word pairs using the worksheet, just as you did for the lesson. The child may want to say the paired words on his own, without repeating them after you. Excellent! Actually, you might encourage him to do so. Allow the child to decide whether or not he wishes to select a turn-taking activity. Some children enjoy doing the worksheet alone. You can even try putting a reinforcer such as a poker chip, raisin, M&M, or penny on each picture that the child correctly completes. Pennies, poker chips, etc., on the pictures allow the child to see how well he is doing. Do not put a reinforcer on a picture the child had difficulty with. After he completes the sheet, go back to the pictures that do not have a reinforcer and practice those. Place a reinforcer on each picture as the child succeeds saying the word pair. Praise the child for a job well done.

Practice Session 1

Practice word pairs using the worksheet. However, this time switch the words *see, say, sew* and *sit* to different rows. In other words, pair each picture in the first row with, for example, the word *sit*. You will say *sit sand, sit sock,* and so on. Use a different first word for rows 2, 3, and 4. Once again the child can select a turn-taking activity or he may choose to do the sheet alone. Pennies, M&Ms, etc., may also be used as in Practice Session 1. Praise the child for a job well done.

Practice Session 2

The child can do Practice Session 3 with or without a turn-taking activity.

This session the child will start by selecting any three pictures on Worksheet 2 for pairing. He will point to each picture and pair that picture with any other word that begins with sssss. He can use *see, say, sit,* and *sew* if he chooses. Or, he may choose to think of his own pairing word, such as "sell." Thus, the child may point to sink, pair it with sell and say, "Sell sink." After he has paired any first three pictures, he selects another three pictures for word pairing. This time he uses a different pairing word, such as "sing," to pair with the picture he has selected. Continue in this fashion, three pictures at a time, until all the pictures on the worksheet have been paired. Praise the child for a job well done.

Practice Session 3

TROUBLESHOOTING

Some children have difficulty remembering to use sssss twice. You can help the child get over this difficulty by saying each word of the pair individually. In other words, you say the first word of the pair and the child repeats that word. Then say the second word of the pair and ask the child to repeat that word. The word pairs for each row of the worksheet are found under Step Two.
Below is an example of how you should present the pairs in Troubleshooting:

You say:	*See*
The child says:	*See*
You say:	*Sun*
The child says:	*Sun*

You can do Step Two and Practice Sessions 1 and 2 with the child. Just remember that the child repeats the first word of the pair before you say the second word of the pair. Praise him for a job well done. When you feel the child is ready, ask him to repeat an entire word pair. If he is successful, do Step 2 and the Practice Sessions as written. If the child has difficulty repeating the word pair, stay in Troubleshooting until he is able to repeat two initial sssss words together.

Do not ask or expect the child to use sssss in conversation yet.

PAIRING FINAL SSSSS SIMPLE WORDS

 ## GOAL

You will teach the child how to pair two words which end with the sssss sound.

  ## MATERIALS

Turn-taking activity
Worksheet 3

 ## LESSON TIME

Approximately 20 minutes

WHAT TO DO

Step One   Review final sssss in simple words in Lesson 6 and pairing initial sssss simple words in Lesson 7. Praise the child for a job well done. Allow him to take a turn at the activity selected. Move on to Step Two. If the child has difficulty using final sssss in simple words, return to Lesson 6. **Do not move on to Step Two until the child is successful at Lesson 6.**

If the child has difficulty using initial sssss in word pairs, continue to do Lesson 7 until the child is successful. *You may, however, also move on to Step Two if the child succeeded in completing Lesson 6.*

⇩   ⇩   ⇩   ⇩   ⇩

Step Two   Your will now help the child pair final sssss simple words. Place Worksheet 3 in front of the child. Each picture on the sheet will be paired with one of the following final sssss words: **is, has, pass, miss**. As you point to the pictures in each row you will say:

First Row:	*is rose, is house, is grass, is goose*
Second Row:	*has bus, has face, has nose, has glass*
Third Row:	*pass mouse, pass kiss, pass dress, pass cactus*
Fourth Row:	*miss moose, miss gas, miss hose, miss nurse*

Begin with the first row. Point to the first picture. Say the paired words. Ask the child to say what you said. Make sure he uses final sssss in each word of the pair. You and the child take turns at the turn-taking activity. Continue if the child pairs without difficulty. See Troubleshooting if the child has difficulty using sssss in both words.

⇩   ⇩   ⇩   ⇩   ⇩

Step Three   Now point to each picture and say the word pairs for each picture in the rest of the row. The child will repeat the word pair for each picture after you. Take turns at the turn-taking activity after you complete the row.

Move on to the second row of pictures. Point and say the word pair for each picture. The child will repeat the word pair for each picture after you. Take turns at the turn-taking activity after you complete the row. Do rows 3 and 4 as you did rows 1 and 2.

Practice the word pairs using the picture sheet just as you did for the lesson. Your child may want to say the paired words on his own, without repeating them after you. Excellent! Actually, you might encourage him to do so.

Practice Session 1

Allow the child to decide whether or not he wishes to select a turn-taking activity. Some children enjoy doing the worksheet alone. You can even try putting a reinforcer such as poker chip, raisin, M&M, or penny on each picture that the child correctly completes. Pennies, poker chips, etc., on the pictures allow the child to see how well he is doing. Do not put a reinforcer on a picture the child had difficulty with. After he completes the sheet, go back to the pictures that do not have a reinforcer and practice those. Place a poker chip or penny, etc., on each picture as the child succeeds saying the word pair. Praise the child for a job well done.

👍 👌 👍 👌 👍

Practice word pairs using the worksheet. However, this time switch the words *is, has, pass, miss* to different rows. In other words, pair each picture in the first row with, for example, the word *miss*. You will say *miss rose, miss house, miss grass, miss goose*. You will use a different first word for rows 2, 3, and 4. Once again the child can select a turn-taking activity if he chooses or do the sheet alone. Pennies, raisins, etc., may also be used as in Practice Session 1. Praise the child for a job well done.

Practice Session 2

👍 👌 👍 👌 👍

The child can do Practice Session 3 with or without a turn-taking activity. This session your child will select any three pictures on Worksheet 3 for pairing. He will point to each picture and pair that picture with any word he selects which ends in sssss. He can use *is, has, pass,* and *miss* if he chooses. Or he may choose to think of his own pairing word which ends in sssss, such as "chase." Thus the child may point to "mouse," pair it with "chase" and say,"Chase mouse." After he has paired the first three pictures, he selects another three pictures for word pairing. This time he uses a different pairing word to pair with the picture. Continue in this fashion, three pictures at a time, until all the pictures on the worksheet have been paired. Praise the child for a job well done.

Practice Session 3

TROUBLESHOOTING

Some children have difficulty remembering to use sssss twice. You can help the child get over this difficulty by saying each word of the pair individually. In other words, you say the first word of the pair and the child repeats that word. Then say the second word of the pair and ask the child to repeat that word. The word pairs for each row of the worksheet are found under Step Two.
Below is an example of how you should present the pairs in Troubleshooting:

You say:	*Is*
The child says:	*Is*
You say:	*Bus*
The child says:	*Bus*

You can do Step Two and Practice Sessions 1 and 2 with the child. Just remember that the child repeats the first word of the pair before you say the second word of the pair. When you feel the child is ready, ask him to repeat an entire word pair. If he is successful, do Step Two and the Practice Sessions as written. If the child has difficulty repeating the word pair, stay in Troubleshooting until he is able to repeat two final sssss words together.

Do not ask or expect the child to use sssss in conversation yet.

MEDIAL SSSS IN SIMPLE WORDS

9

GOAL

You will teach the child to use sssss in the middle of words.

MATERIALS

Turn-taking Activity
Worksheet 4

LESSON TIME

Approximately 20 minutes

WHAT TO DO

Step One   Review Lessons 7 and 8. Praise the child for a job well done. Allow him to take a turn at the activity selected.

⇩   ⇩   ⇩   ⇩   ⇩

Step Two   Before you begin working on medial sssss, a word of explanation is in order. Sssss in the middle of words is produced either as an initial sssss sound or as a final sssss sound. For example, sssss in the word "castle" is produced as an initial sssss. The child will be instructed to say "ca," then "stle." However, sssss in the word "basket" is said as a final sssss. The child will be asked to say "bas," then "ket." Try to ignore how a word is spelled, for this lesson, and concentrate on how the word is said.

⇩   ⇩   ⇩   ⇩   ⇩

Step Three   Look at Worksheet 4. Look at the right-hand corner of each picture. You should see either an "I" or an "F" on each picture. If a picture has the letter "I," then the sssss for that picture is produced as an initial sssss sound. If a picture has the letter "F," then the sssss for that picture is said as a final sssss sound. As an additional guide, below are words for Worksheet 4 listed as either Produced As Initial or Produced As Final. I have listed them as they will be said by you and repeated by the child.

PRODUCED AS INITIAL			PRODUCED AS FINAL		
bicycle	*bi*	*sikle*	basket	*bas*	*ket*
whistle	*wi*	*sil*	grasshopper	*grass*	*hopper*
pencil	*pen*	*sil*	rooster	*roos*	*ter*
eraser	*era*	*ser*	baseball	*base*	*ball*
castle	*ca*	*sil*	toaster	*toas*	*ter*
present	*pre*	*zent*	bracelet	*brace*	*let*
dinosaur	*dino*	*sore*	costume	*cos*	*tume*
tricycle	*tri*	*sickle*	classroom	*class*	*room*

You will now help the child use the medial sssss sound in words. Place Worksheet 4 in front of the child. You name the first picture. Remember to say each syllable clearly so that the child can hear with which syllable the sssss will be said. The child names the picture after you. Allow the child to take a turn at the turn-taking activity selected, after he has named three pictures after you. You also take a turn.

You continue naming and taking turns at the activity until you and the child have named each picture. Remember to take turns at the selected activity. Review the sheet a second time, taking turns at the selected activity. Praise the child for a job well done. See Troubleshooting if the child lisps when repeating each word or has difficulty repeating sssss in simple words

PRACTICE SESSIONS

Practice medial words using the picture sheet just as you did for the lesson. Allow the child to decide whether or not he wishes to select a turn-taking activity. Or, the child may decide to place a reinforcer such as a poker chip, raisin, M&M, or penny on each picture that he correctly names. Do not allow the child to put a poker chip, raisin, etc., on a picture he said incorrectly. After he completes the sheet, go back to the pictures which do not have a reinforcer on them and practice those. Place a reinforcer on each picture as the child successfully says the medial sssss word. Praise the child for a job well done.

Your child can do Practice Session 2 with or without a turn-taking activity. This session the child will select any three pictures. He will point to each picture and name it using a correct sssss. Praise him for a job well done. The child will continue in this fashion until all the pictures on the worksheet have been named.

TROUBLESHOOTING

Some children have difficulty making the transition from sssss immediately to the next sound in the same word. You can help the child get over this difficulty by saying each syllable of the word individually. In other words, you say the first syllable of the word and the child repeats that syllable. Then say the second syllable of the word and ask the child to repeat that syllable. The breakdown of syllables can be found under Step Three. Complete Worksheet 4 with the child repeating one syllable at a time, for each word, after you. Remember to take turns at the turn-taking activity after each group of three pictures named in this syllable-by-syllable presentation. Praise the child for a job well done. Stay in Troubleshooting until the child is able to say medial sssss in a word without a syllable-by-syllable breakdown.

You can do Practice Sessions 1 and 2 with the child. Just remember that the child repeats each syllable separately after you until you feel he is ready to use medial sssss without a separation of syllables.

Do not ask or expect the child to use sssss in conversation yet.

INITIAL SSSSS IN SIMPLE SENTENCES

10

GOAL

You will teach the child to begin using initial sssss in simple sentences.

MATERIALS

Worksheet 2
Turn-taking Activity

LESSON TIME

Approximately 20 minutes

WHAT TO DO

Step One   Review pairing initial and final sssss simple words and medial words in Lessons 7, 8, and 9. Praise the child for a job well done. Allow him to take a turn at the activity selected. Move on to Step Two. If the child has difficulty using initial sssss in pairs, return to Lesson 7. **Do not move on to Step Two until the child is successful at Lesson 7**.

If the child has difficulty pairing final sssss simple words or with medial sssss in simple words, continue to do those lessons until the child is successful. *You may, however, also move on to Step Two if the child succeeded in completing Lesson 7.*

⇩   ⇩   ⇩   ⇩   ⇩

Step Two   You will now help the child use the word pairs of Lesson 7 in simple sentences. Place Worksheet 2 in front of the child. You will work a row at a time as you did in Lesson 7. (Some of the sentences will not make sense. That is okay. Right now our goal is for the child to begin using the sssss sound in sentences. Actually, you and the child can have fun laughing at the silliness of some of the sentences.) Each sentence will begin with the word "I" plus a verb. You will say the following at each row:

First Row: *I see sand. I see a sock. I see soap. I see a sun.*
Second Row: *I say seal. I say saw. I say seven. I say soup.*
Third Row: *I sew a safe. I sew a sail. I sew a suit. I sew a sofa.*
Fourth Row: *I sit on a sink. I sit on salt. I sit on a saddle. I sit on soda.*

Begin with the first row of pictures. Point to the first picture. Say the sentence for that picture. Ask the child to say what you said. Make sure he uses initial sssss in each word starting with sssss. Praise the child for a job well done. Take turns at the turn-taking activity. Continue if the child repeats the sentence without difficulty. See Troubleshooting if the child has difficulty using sssss in simple sentences.

⇩   ⇩   ⇩   ⇩   ⇩

Step Three   Now point and say the sentence for each picture in the rest of the row. The child will repeat the sentence for each picture after you. Praise the child for a job well done. Take turns at the turn-taking activity after the child completes the row.

Move on to the second row of pictures. Point and say the sentence for each picture. The child will repeat the sentence for each picture after you. Praise the child and take turns at the activity. Do rows 3 and 4 in the same way.

PRACTICE SESSIONS

Practice the simple sentences using the worksheet just as you did for the lesson. Your child may want to say the sentences on his own, without repeating them after you. Excellent! Actually, you might encourage him to do so. Allow the child to decide whether or not he wishes to select a turn-taking activity, or use reinforcers such as pennies, poker chips, etc. Once the child has completed the sheet, go back and practice any sentences he had trouble with.

Practice Session 1

Practice sentences using the worksheet. However, this time switch the *I* + verb (*see, say, sew, sit*) to different rows. In other words, say each picture in the first row with, for example, *I sit* instead of *I see*. You will say *I sit on sand, I sit on a sock, I sit on a soap, I sit on a sun.* Switch *I see* to another row, such as row 2, *I say* to row 3, and *I sew* to row 4. You can use any first two words with any row you or the child wishes. Once again the child can select a turn-taking activity if he chooses or do the sheet alone. Pennies, poker chips, raisins, M&Ms, etc., may also be used. Or, since this is the last time you will be using this worksheet, the child can color, apply stickers to, or draw a happy face on each picture for which sssss was correctly said. Do not allow the child to color or put a sticker on a picture he said incorrectly. After he completes the sheet, go back to the pictures that are not colored or do not have a sticker. Practice those pictures. Allow the child to color or put a sticker or happy face on each picture as he succeeds in saying the sentence correctly. Praise him for a job well done.

Practice Session 2

TROUBLESHOOTING

Some children have difficulty remembering to use sssss in a sentence. You can help the child get over this difficulty by saying each word of the sentence individually. In other words, you say *I* and the child repeats *I* Next say "see," which the child repeats. Last, say the picture name, such as "sand," which the child repeats. Praise the child for a job well done.

Stay on the first picture. This time ask the child to repeat "I see." Praise the child for a job well done. Now ask him to repeat "sand." Praise him again. Tell the child that this time he will say the whole sentence after you. You slowly say, "I see sand." Ask the child to repeat what you just said. Praise him for a job well done. Complete the first row in this way. Return to Step Two of this lesson once the child repeats each simple sentence in its entirety, in the first row, using correct sssss. Remember to take turns at the turn-taking activity. If the child has difficulty repeating the entire sentence, stay with "I see," which he repeats, then "sand," which he repeats. Complete the worksheet in this way. Reintroduce the entire sentence once you feel the child is ready. Praise the child frequently and take turns at the activity. The child will be ready to do Step Two of this lesson once he can repeat an entire simple sentence for each picture in the first row.

Do not ask or expect the child to use sssss in conversation yet.

FINAL SSSSS IN SIMPLE SENTENCES

11

 GOAL

You will teach the child to begin using final sssss in simple sentences.

  MATERIALS

Worksheet 3
Turn-taking Activity

 LESSON TIME

Approximately 20 minutes

WHAT TO DO

Step One   Review pairing final sssss simple words in Lesson 8, medial sssss in words in Lesson 9, and initial sssss in simple sentences in Lesson 10. Praise the child for a job well done. Allow him to take a turn at the activity selected. Move on to Step Two. If the child has difficulty pairing <u>final</u> sssss simple words, return to Lesson 8. **Do not move on to Step Two until the child is successful at Lesson 8.**

If the child has difficulty using <u>medial</u> sssss in simple words (Lesson 9) or <u>initial</u> sssss in simple sentences (Lesson 10) continue to do those lessons until the child is successful. *You may, however, also move on to Step Two if the child succeeded in completing Lesson 8.*

⇩   ⇩   ⇩   ⇩   ⇩

Step Two   You will now help the child use the word pairs of Lesson 8, in simple sentences. Place Worksheet 4 in front of the child. You will work a row at a time as you did in Lesson 8. (Some of the sentences will not make sense. That is okay. Right now our goal is for the child to begin using the sssss sound in sentences.)

Look at the worksheet. You will say the following:

First Row: *Here is a rose. Here is a house. Here is grass. Here is a goose.*
Second Row: *He has a bus. He has a face. He has a nose. He has a glass.*
Third Row: *I pass a mouse. I pass a kiss. I pass a dress. I pass a cactus.*
Fourth Row: *I miss a moose. I miss gas. I miss a hose. I miss a nurse.*

Begin with the first row of pictures. Point to the first picture. Say the sentence for that picture. Ask the child to say what you said. Make sure he uses final sssss in each word ending with sssss. Praise the child for a job well done. Take turns at the turn-taking activity. Continue if the child repeats the sentence without difficulty. See Troubleshooting if the child has difficulty using sssss in simple sentences.

⇩   ⇩   ⇩   ⇩   ⇩

Step Three   Now point and say the sentence for each picture in the rest of the row. The child will repeat the sentence for each picture after you. Praise the child for a job well done. Take turns at the turn-taking activity. Do rows 3 and 4 in the same way.

PRACTICE SESSIONS

Practice the simple sentences using the worksheet, just as you did for the lesson. The child may want to say the paired words on his own, without repeating them after you. Excellent! Actually, you might encourage him to do so. Allow the child to decide whether or not he wishes to select a turn-taking activity or use reinforcers (pennies, poker chips, etc.). Once the child has completed the worksheet, go back and practice any sentences he had trouble with.

Practice Session 1

Practice sentences using the worksheet. However, this time switch the first two words of the sentences with the other rows. In other words, say each picture in the first row with *I miss* instead of *Here is*. You will say *I miss a rose, I miss a house, I miss grass, I miss a goose*. Switch *Here is* to another row, such as row 2, *He has* to row 3, and *I pass* to row 4. You can use any first two words with any row you or the child wishes. Once again the child can select a turn-taking activity if he chooses or do the worksheet alone. Reinforcers (pennies, M&Ms, Skittles, etc.) may also be used. Since this is the last time we will be using this worksheet, the child can color in, put a sticker on, or draw a happy face on each picture for which sssss was correctly said. Do not allow the child to color in, put a sticker on, or draw a happy face on a picture he said incorrectly. After he completes the sheet, go back to the pictures which are not colored or do not have a sticker or happy face. Practice those pictures. Allow the child to color in, put a sticker on, or draw a happy face on each picture as he succeeds in saying the sentence correctly. Praise him for a job well done.

Practice Session 2

TROUBLESHOOTING

Some children have difficulty remembering to use sssss in a sentence. You can help the child get over this difficulty by saying each word of the sentence individually. In other words, you say *Here* and the child repeats *Here*. Next, say *is a* which the child repeats. Last say the picture name, such as *rose*, which the child repeats. Praise the child for a job well done.

Stay on the first picture. This time ask the child to repeat *Here is*. Praise him for a job well done. Now ask him to repeat *a rose*. Praise him again. Tell the child that this time he will say the whole sentence after you. You slowly say *Here is a rose*. Ask the child to repeat what you just said. Praise him for a job well done. Complete the first row in this way. Return to Step Two of this lesson once the child repeats each sentence in its entirety, in the first row, using correct sssss in a sentence. Remember to take turns at the turn-taking activity. If the child has difficulty repeating the entire sentence, stay with *Here is*, which he repeats, then *a rose*, which he repeats. Complete the sheet in this way. Reintroduce the **entire sentence,** *Here is a rose*, once you feel the child is ready. The child will be ready to do Step Two of this lesson once he can repeat a simple sentence, in its entirety, for each picture in the first row.

Do not ask or expect the child to use sssss in conversation yet.

SSSSS IN BLENDS

 GOAL

You will teach the child to use *st, sk, sl, sp, sm, sn, sw, str, spr,* and *scr* in words.

Note: Not all the blends will be taught in the lesson. Half are taught in the lesson and the other half are taught in Practice Session 1. If you are a student, you may want to break this lesson into two therapy sessions. If you do so, Practice Session 1 would become another therapy session. If you decide to make Practice Session 1 a therapy session, instruct the parent to practice Worksheet 5 at home. After you complete Worksheet 6 in the next therapy session, instruct the parent to practice Worksheet 6 at home. Instruct the parent to do Practice Sessions 2 and 3 as written.

 MATERIALS

Worksheets 5 and 6
Turn-taking Activity

 LESSON TIME

Approximately 30 minutes

WHAT TO DO

Step One   Review medial words and initial and final sssss in simple sentences in Lessons 9, 10, and 11. Praise the child for a job well done. Allow him to take a turn at the activity selected. Move on to Step Two.

If the child has difficulty using medial words or initial or final sssss in simple sentences, continue to do those lessons which he is having difficulty with until he is successful. *You may, however, also move on to Step Two if you feel the child is ready.*

⇩   ⇩   ⇩   ⇩   ⇩

Step Two   This step can make learning sssss in blends fun. You will now try kinesthetic cuing. This means that the child will "feel" and say the sound at the same time. The first thing you need to do is practice kinesthetic cuing on yourself. Place the index finger of your right hand on the wrist of your left arm. As you say sssss, simultaneously move your index finger up your left arm to your shoulder. You will need to stretch out the sssss sound for the length of time it takes your finger to move from your wrist to your shoulder. (The finger movement up your arm should take about four seconds.) As soon as you reach your shoulder, jump your index finger to your mouth and say the rest of the word. Let's use the word "step" to practice. Place your right index finger on your left wrist. Start moving your index finger up your arm as you say "sssss." When you get to your shoulder, jump your finger to your mouth and say the rest of the word "tep." Practice kinesthetic cuing a few more times using the word "step" or any other word on Worksheet 5. When you feel you are ready to do kinesthetic cuing with the child move on to Step Three.

You will now use kinesthetic cuing with the child. Look at the first picture on Worksheet 5. Place your index finger on the child's wrist. Tell the child that he will "feel" the sssss sound "stretch" on his arm. Proceed to say "sssss" as you move your finger from the child's wrist to his shoulder. When you reach his shoulder jump to his mouth and say the rest of the word "tep." Now do the same thing with the child saying the word with you. Praise the child for a job well done. Repeat the kinesthetic cuing for the word "step." Do a few more pictures in this way. Remember to take turns at the turn-taking activity. When you feel your child is ready, move on to #1 below. See Troubleshooting if your child is having difficulty "stretching" the sssss and then combining it with the rest of the word.

1. Instead of placing your finger on the child's wrist, place it halfway up his arm. Now as you move your finger up the child's arm, the sssss will be stretched for only two seconds. When your finger reaches the child's shoulder it will jump to his mouth, at which time he will say the rest of the word. Do a few pictures in this way. Praise the child for a job well done and take turns at the turn-taking activity. When you feel the child is ready, move to #2 below. If the child has difficulty saying the word with only a two-second "stretch" of the sssss, continue to do the words, stretching the sssss for four seconds. Come back to the two-second stretch when you feel the child is ready.

2. Demonstrate the following for the child. Place your index finger on your shoulder. Move your finger from your shoulder to your mouth as you say the complete word, "sweat." The sssss should NOT be stretched and should blend into the rest of the word. Now tell the child it is his turn. Place your index finger on the child's shoulder. Tell him to say the word "sweat" with you. Move your finger from his shoulder to his mouth as you say the word together. Do the same for a few more pictures. After a few successes, praise the child and move to #3 below. If the child has difficulty saying the word without "stretching," return to #1 above.

3. The child will now say the word without kinesthetic cuing. Tell the child that now he will say the pictures without "feeling" the sssss. Point to the picture and say the word. The child repeats the word after you. Praise the child. Do all the words on the worksheet this way. Remember to take turns at the turn-taking activity. If the child has difficulty saying the words without kinesthetic cuing, return to #2 above.

PRACTICE SESSIONS

Practice Session 1

Practice sssss in blends using Worksheet 6. Allow the child to decide whether or not he wishes to select a turn-taking activity or use reinforcers (pennies, poker chips, etc.). Before you start, think back to Step Three of this lesson. Was the child able to repeat the sssss in blends words without "stretching" the sssss? If the answer is yes, the child should be able to repeat these new words without hearing you exaggerate sssss. Complete this sheet, saying the words as you would normally.

Continue to use a "stretched" sssss when naming these pictures if the child needs to hear a "stretched" sssss in order to say the word with the sssss sound. Try to gradually reduce the length of the "stretched" sssss as you do the worksheet. Ask the child to say the words just the way you say them.

Practice Session 2

Worksheets 5 and 6 will be used for this practice session. Allow the child to decide whether or not he wishes to use a turn-taking activity and/or reinforcers (raisins, poker chips, etc.). Before you start, tell the child that you will be listening for his good sssss. Point to a picture on one of the worksheets. Say the word as you normally would, without "stretching" the sssss. Ask the child to say what you just said. Praise the child. He can put a reinforcer on the picture. Point to another picture, name it, and ask the child to say what you just said. The child can continue to put reinforcers on the pictures correctly named. A turn at the turn-taking activity can be taken after three or four pictures are named. Remember to praise the child for a job well done.

Practice Session 3

Worksheets 5 and 6 will be used for this session. Allow the child to select a turn-taking activity if he wishes. He may color the pictures, draw a happy face, or place a sticker, raisin, penny, etc., on each picture of each worksheet. Tell the child that today *he* will point to the pictures. Tell him that you will be listening for his good sssss sound. Ask the child to point to a picture and name it. Praise him for a job well done. If he likes he may color or draw a happy face on each picture. Or, if he is using pennies, stickers, etc., allow him to place one on the picture if it was correctly named. Ask the child to point to three more pictures and name each. Praise the child and take turns at the turn-taking activity if one was selected. If the child has difficulty naming the picture, you name it and ask him to say what you said. Do not allow the child to color, draw a happy face, or put a reinforcer on a picture he has difficulty with. Instead, after the child has completed the worksheets, go back to those pictures which are not colored or do not have a sticker, raisin, etc. Ask the child to name those pictures again. He can color, draw a happy face on, or put a reinforcer on each picture named correctly. Remember to praise the child for a job well done.

TROUBLESHOOTING:

Some children have difficulty blending two consonants together. You can help the child by separating the sssss from the rest of the word. Look at the first picture on Worksheet 5. Instead of saying, "Step," you will say " *Sssss,*" which the child repeats, then, " *tep,*" which the child repeats. Praise the child for a job well done. Say each word in the first row in this way—you say the sssss, the child says sssss, you say the rest of the word, the child says the rest of the word. Praise the child for a job well done.**

After you and the child have finished the first row, go back to the first picture in that row and point to it. You will say this word again. But this time do not separate the sssss from the rest of the word. Instead, exaggerate the sssss by lengthening it, and then say the rest of the word. In other words, you say "sssssstep." Ask the child to say what you just said. If the child has difficulty doing this on his own, help him by saying the word together, with an exaggerated sssss. Then ask the child to say it again by himself. Once the child is able to repeat a row with an exaggerated sssss, return to Step Three #2 of this lesson.

**You may choose to do another row, or the entire worksheet, in this way—separating the sssss from the rest of the word. That is fine. When you feel the child is ready, continue as instructed in Troubleshooting.

Do not ask or expect the child to use sssss in conversation yet.

SENTENCES USING INITIAL, MEDIAL, AND FINAL SSSSS AND SSSSS IN BLENDS

13

GOAL

The child will use sssss, in any position, in sentences.

MATERIALS

Worksheets 7, 8, and 9

LESSON TIME

15 minutes

WHAT TO DO

Step One   You and the child should sit next to each other. Look at Worksheet 7. Each picture has writing under it. Tell the child that you will be reading a story together. As the child looks at the first picture you will read the first sentence under the picture. Read the sentence slowly with a slight exaggeration of every sssss sound. Ask the child to repeat the sentence you just said. Remind him to say all his sssss sounds. Listen carefully as the child says the sentence. It is not unusual for children to forget to use the sssss. If the child forgets to use sssss in any word, wait until he has finished the sentence. Tell the child he forgot to use his sssss sound in the word _____. Ask him to repeat the word using his sssss sound. After he has correctly repeated the word, say the same sentence again. Ask the child to repeat what you just said. Praise him for a job well done. Complete the worksheet with the child, reading no more than one sentence at a time.

⇩   ⇩   ⇩   ⇩   ⇩

Step Two   Look at Worksheet 8 with the child. Do this worksheet just as you did Worksheet 7 in Step One. Remember to frequently praise the child.

Sit next to the child. Look at Worksheet 9 with the child. Do this worksheet just as you did Worksheets 7 and 8 of the Lesson. Remember to praise the child for a job well done.

Practice Session 1

Sit next to the child. Show the child Worksheets 7, 8, and 9. Ask him to pick the worksheet he wishes to do first. Do this worksheet just as you had done in the lesson. Do the same for the other two worksheets. The child can color in the pictures if he wishes to do so. Remember to praise him frequently.

Practice Session 2

Sit next to the child. Show the child worksheets 7, 8, and 9. Ask him questions about the worksheets' stories. Make sure your questions require a sentence answer from the child and not a "yes" or "no" answer. For example, ask questions such as: What happened ...; Why is ...; How did ...; etc. You can also elicit speech by saying, "Tell me about ..." Watch the child's mouth carefully as he answers. Make sure he uses his correct sssss. If he lisps, tell him on what word he lisped. Ask him to say the word again using his sssss sound. Praise him for a job well done.

Practice Session 3

Do not ask or expect the child to use sssss in conversation yet.

51

USING SSSSS WHILE PLAYING

 ## GOAL

The child will use sssss in conversation for a limited period of time in a controlled play environment.

 ## MATERIALS

Reinforcers:
Small items that can be placed in a cup, such as poker chips, pennies, popcorn, raisins, M&M's, etc. You will need about 15 of the item you selected (example: 15 pennies). The child will need to earn a certain number of reinforcers (poker chips, pennies, M&Ms, etc.) in order to get a reward.

Rewards:
Rewards such as a candy bar, ice cream cone, stickers, or any item which will motivate the child. If you use M&Ms, raisins, or other small food as reinforcers, they can be used as the reward. In other words, he gets to eat all the M&Ms he won. **The reward is given at the end of the lesson.**

Conversational Activities:
You will need an activity that allows you and the child to talk with each other. When playing with the child he should, ideally, dominate the conversation. Avoid doing activities during which you know the child rarely talks. If the child does not talk much while playing, you should try to engage him in conversation about what is happening as you play. Below are examples of activities that are appropriate for this lesson. See Appendix C for more ideas.

- Barbie dolls
- Race cars with gas station or other props you can use to encourage your child to talk while playing.
- Playing school, house, supermarket, astronaut, cowboys, etc. Your child may choose to play with or without dolls or action figures.
- Read a book. You and the child can take turns reading a book. Keep in mind that your child does not have to know how to read. Telling a story by looking at pictures in a book is an excellent activity for nonreaders.

 ## LESSON TIME

Approximately 30 minutes

WHAT TO DO

Step One   Allow the child to select an activity along the lines of the examples given under Materials. Tell the child that as you play together you will be listening for his good sssss sound. Tell him that he will earn a chip (or penny or M&M depending on what you have selected) each time he says his good sssss when talking. If he wins three chips he gets the _____ (name the reward) after the session is over. In other words, the child needs to say sssss correctly a minimum of three times during this entire lesson.

⇩   ⇩   ⇩   ⇩   ⇩

Step Two   The sssss is common enough to appear in every sentence one or more times. Listen carefully to the child as he talks. Each time he uses sssss correctly praise him, tell him he gets a chip for using his sssss, and allow him to place one chip in his cup. As you play, give him frequent reminders that you are listening for his good sssss sound when he talks. If the child says an sssss word but forgets to use sssss and lisps instead, do the following:

1. Ask the child to stop playing.
2. Ask the child to look at you.
3. Tell the child that he forgot to use his good sssss in the word _____.
4. Ask the child to say _____ with a good sssss. Praise him after he says the word correctly but do not give him a chip.
5. Remind the child to use his good sssss when he talks so that he can get a chip.

If the child uses sssss for words that do not have an sssss sound, see Troubleshooting.

**It is important to understand that using a new sound in conversation can be a difficult and slow process. This is normal and okay. Your job will be to help the child along so that he gradually uses sssss more frequently. It is of utmost importance to be patient and have realistic expectations. Your goal is to challenge him without frustrating him or yourself.

There will be five practice sessions for Lesson 14. It is recommended that the child complete one practice session every day. Doing a practice session every day will help the child get used to using sssss in conversation, which will be the goal of the last session, Lesson 15. As you do the practice sessions you will gradually be requiring the child to remember to use sssss more often. You will do this by slowly increasing the number of reinforcers (pennies, chips, etc.) he will need to earn a reward.

👍 👌 👍 👌 👍

You will need reinforcers and a reward. See Materials in the lesson for ideas.

Practice Session 1

Allow the child to select a toy along the lines of that which was selected for the lesson. Tell the child that you will be listening for his good sssss sound while he plays with you. Remind the child that he will win a penny (or whatever reinforcer is selected) each time he says his good sssss sound in his words. Tell him that today he will need to win five _____ (name the reinforcer) to win a _____ (name the reward selected). He gets the reward when the session is over.

Play with the child for about 30 minutes. Follow the instructions under Step Two of the lesson.

👍 👌 👍 👌 👍

You will follow the same instructions for this practice session as you did for Practice Session 1. The child will still need five pennies, chips, etc., to get a reward.

Practice Session 2

👍 👌 👍 👌 👍

The instructions are the same. However, you will tell the child that this time he will need eight _____ (name the reinforcer) in order to get a_____ (name the reward) at the end of the session.

Practice Session 3

👍 👌 👍 👌 👍

Once again the instructions are the same. Only the number of reinforcers needed for a reward will change. During this session the child will need 10 reinforcers in order to win a reward at the end of the session.

Practice Session 4

Practice Session 5

Same as Practice Session 4.

TROUBLESHOOTING

Some children overgeneralize using their new sound. In other words, they are not sure which words should have an sssss sound so they use sssss on all words or they randomly use sssss. For example, a child might say ssssbig. You can help the child get over this difficulty by doing the following:

1. Tell the child that not every word has a sssss sound. "big" does not have a sssss sound. Tell the child we say "big."
2. Ask the child to repeat the word correctly—"Big."

Do not ask or expect the child to use sssss in conversation yet.

USING SSSS IN CONVERSATION

☆ GOAL

The child will learn to use sssss in conversation all the time.

MATERIALS

- 60 pennies
- 10 nickels
- Two clear cups. One cup should have a picture of a happy face drawn on it.
- Prize which the child will earn. The prize need not be expensive. The child should select the prize. Examples: a special doll or action figure, game, toy, a trip to the movies, clothing, etc. If you are not the parent doing this program, ask that the parent purchase the reward upon completion of the program.

⏱ LESSON TIME

Approximately one month

WHAT TO DO

Parents using this program should follow the instructions below beginning with Step One. If you are not the parent, look in Appendix B for a duplicate to this lesson. Copy Appendix B and give it to the parent to use. Go over the entire lesson with the parent. After you and the parent have gone over the lesson together, hand the parent the lesson in Appendix B to take home. The parent will complete this lesson at home. Request that the parent bring the child to see you once or twice weekly so that you can monitor his progress.

There is a certificate at the end of the lesson. Sign and give the child the certificate after he has successfully completed this lesson.

⇩   ⇩   ⇩   ⇩   ⇩

Step One

Place the 60 pennies in the clear cup without the happy face. Place the 10 nickels next to the cup.

Show the nickels and the cup with the 60 pennies to the child. Tell the child he is going to try to win all the pennies that are in the cup. Tell him that he will win a penny each time he uses his good sssss when he talks. Each time he wins a penny he will put it into the happy face cup. After he wins all the pennies and nickels he will win a prize of his choice.

Ask the child what prize he would like to win. You might want to take a trip to a store so that he can show you what he wants. The prize should be something the child will be motivated to win. As you do Lesson 15 you will be frequently reminding the child what he is working to win. If the child has a picture of what he wants, you can tape the picture on the second cup instead of drawing a happy face on it.

⇩   ⇩   ⇩   ⇩   ⇩

Step Two

It is very important that you monitor, or listen carefully to, the child whenever he is speaking. The sssss occurs frequently in English. The more often you catch and correct the child's errors, the faster he will learn to use sssss in conversation. As you start the penny program, realize that the child will lisp more often than he uses sssss. This is normal. He will gradually replace the lisp with sssss as you correct his errors and reinforce his use of sssss with praise and the earning of pennies. Once the child has earned all his pennies, he will be ready for Step Three. If you find it too difficult to monitor the child throughout the entire day, you can start out by correcting or reinforcing correct use of sssss during specific periods, such as during mealtimes, for the first couple of days. Increase your monitoring from mealtimes to an entire half day, for no more than two more days. Your next increase will be to monitor the child throughout as much of the day as possible.

If the child is in preschool or daycare for most of the day, speak to the person caring for the child. Tell this person that the child is learning to use his sssss sound in conversation. Give the caretaker a small notebook. Ask her to watch the child when he talks. Whenever she hears and sees him using his correct sssss she should praise him and record his using sssss by drawing a star in the notebook for each time he used sssss. If the child used sssss five times, then the notebook should have five stars drawn in it. When you pick the child up ask the caretaker how he did using sssss during the day. Look at the small notebook, with the child, and together count the number of stars the caretaker made. Praise the child for using sssss. When you get home, place a penny in the cup for each star earned during the day.

WHAT TO DO WHEN THE CHILD CORRECTLY USES SSSSS

As you begin Lesson 15 you will need to give the child a penny **each time** he correctly uses sssss, **on his own,** when talking. As he begins to use sssss more often on his own, you will start to give him pennies less frequently. In other words, as he gets better at using sssss, challenge him subtly by giving him a penny after a few words of correct sssss. As time goes on and he uses sssss more often, you will give him a penny only after he has spoken over a period of a couple hours without lisping. As you get down to the last 10 pennies, you should be giving him a penny for correct sssss no more than three times a day.
How do you know if you are giving too few or too many pennies a day? The following will help you gauge how well you are challenging the child with the penny program:

Two to three weeks after starting the penny program, the child should have earned 30 to 40 pennies and should be using sssss, in conversation, about 50 percent of the time.

Four to five weeks after starting the penny program, the child should have earned all the pennies and should be using sssss, in conversation, at least 80 percent of the time.

It is also very important to praise the child. You can praise the child by saying, "Very good! You remembered to say your sssss sound. You said, _____ (repeat the sssss word your child said correctly)." The child will enjoy placing the penny in the cup by himself. He will also enjoy looking in the cup to see how many pennies he has; looking in the cup is a good way for the child to **see** how he is doing. You can also count the chips with him every now and then. He will be pleased to count how many pennies he has earned.

WHAT TO DO WHEN THE CHILD LISPS IN CONVERSATION

As you start the penny program, expect that the child will lisp more often than he will use his correct sssss. When you hear his lisp, say, "You forgot to use your sssss. Let's say _____ (name the word which was lisped) using a good sssss sound." Say the word and ask your child to repeat it correctly (do not give him a penny). Praise the child and say, "Remember to say your sssss when you talk so you can win pennies. You don't get pennies when you forget to say sssss."

WHAT TO DO IF THE CHILD PURPOSELY SAYS A SSSSS WORD AND WANTS A PENNY

The child will be eager to earn pennies. As a result he may approach you and say, out of the blue, a word he knows contains sssss. He may remind you to give him a chip for saying sssss. Praise him for saying a good sssss. You may give him a chip the first couple of times he does this. After the first couple of times, tell him that from now on he gets a penny only when he is talking, and not for thinking of an sssss word to tell you.

WHAT TO DO IF THE CHILD ATTACHES SSSSS TO WORDS THAT DO NOT HAVE A SSSSS SOUND

Some children overgeneralize when learning when to use their sssss sound. In other words, they are not sure which words have an sssss sound so they use sssss on all words or randomly use sssss. For example, a child might say "ssssbig." You can help the child get over this difficulty by doing the following:

1. Tell the child there is no sssss in *big*. Tell him we say *big*.
2. Ask the child to repeat the word correctly —*big*.

⇩　　⇩　　⇩　　⇩　　⇩

Step Three　This step is designed to help make the child more aware of those times he may still lisp. Once the child has earned all 60 pennies, he will be ready to earn nickels. Unlike pennies which could only be won, nickels can be won or lost. In other words, when the child correctly uses sssss for a few hours he earns a nickel and places it with the pennies in the happy face cup. However, if he lisps, he has to take the nickel out of the happy face cup and return it to the original cup.

Congratulate the child for working so hard and winning all his pennies. Tell him that he is almost ready to win his prize. Remove all the pennies from the happy face cup. Place 10 nickels in the empty penny cup. Show the nickels to the child and tell him that when all the nickels are in the happy face cup he will get his prize. Tell him he wins a nickel for using his sssss just like when he won pennies. But, if he forgets to use his sssss, he has to take a nickel out of the happy face cup and put it back in the other cup. Show him how this works by saying and doing the following:

1. "Let's say you're talking and you use sssss a lot. You win a nickel." (Place a nickel in the happy face cup.)

2. "But let's say you're talking and you forget to use sssss and say 'thun' instead of 'sun.' If you say 'thun' I have to take one nickel out of the happy face cup and put it back with the other nickels. (Take a nickel out of the happy face cup.) But if you remember to use your good sssss again, you can win back the nickel."

3. "Remember to use your sssss so that you don't have to lose any nickels."

4. Write down each sssss word the child incorrectly says. At the end of the day go over the list with the child. Say, "Today you forgot to use your sssss for the words I wrote on this paper. We need to practice these words so that tomorrow you will say them correctly and you will not lose a nickel." Then ask him to say each word correctly five times in a row.

It is normal for the child to lose and earn nickels over the course of a few days. Each time a nickel is lost, ask the child to say the word correctly. Remind him to think about using his good sssss so he will not have to lose nickels.

The child should finish the nickels and sssss program once he uses sssss 100% of the time. There is a certificate at the end of the lesson. Sign and give it to him after he has successfully completed this lesson. Also, the child can have the reward he has worked hard to earn.

Certificate of Achievement

This Certifies That

_____

has Successfully Completed

the "S" Program

on this _____ day of _____, _____.

Great Job!

Mirla G. Raz

Mirla G. Raz, M.Ed., C.C.C.

POSTLESSON

MAKING SURE THE CHILD CONTINUES TO USE THE SSSSS SOUND CORRECTLY

Congratulations to you and the child for having successfully corrected his lisp! Before you put this manual away, however, I would like to leave you with a few suggestions and words of advice regarding the child's newly learned sound. If you are a parent, read the information below. If you are a student, professional, or anyone other than the parent, please go over what is written below with the parent.

- First, over the next few days give the child frequent praise for using his good sssss sound. Be generous with praise.
- Second, be on guard for an occasional lisp. If the child slips and lisps, bring the error to his attention. Gently tell him that he forgot to use his sssss when he said _____. Ask him to repeat the word with his sssss sound.

If you notice a gradual increase in lisping I suggest that you begin a motivational program to get the child back on track. For instance, tell him that each morning he will get five nickels in his happy face cup. Tell him he will lose a nickel each time he forgets to use his sssss sound. He must have at least one nickel left in his cup at the end of the day in order to get a reward (such as ice cream, candy, watch a favorite TV program, etc.). After a day or two of getting rewards, reduce the nickels in his happy face cup to three. By reducing the number of nickels you are requiring him to make fewer errors in order to win a reward at the end of the day. Within a few days the child should be back on track.

WORKSHEETS

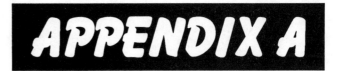

The worksheets in this Appendix are intended to be removed. Remove each worksheet as indicated in the appropriate lesson. Since the worksheets will be reused in other lessons, do not discard worksheets until indicated in the lesson.

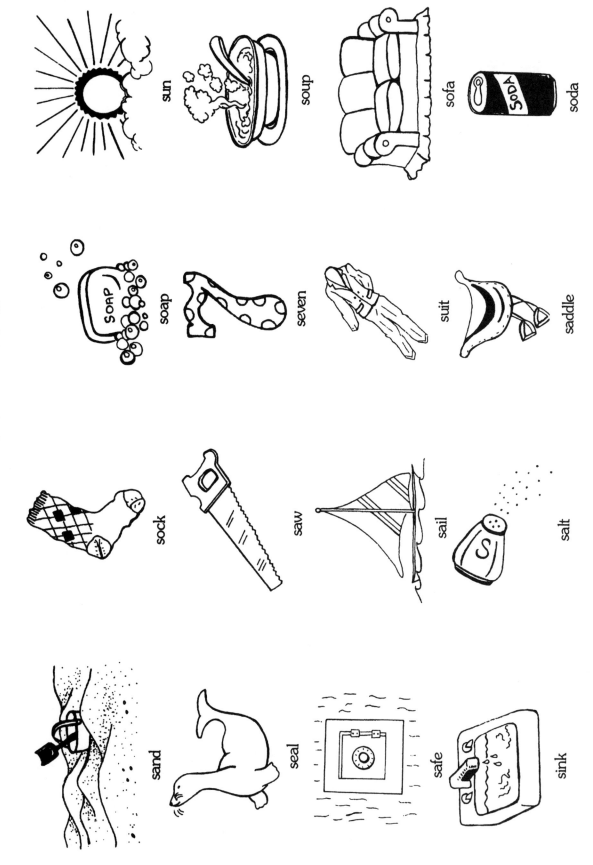

sun

soup

sofa

soda

soap

seven

suit

saddle

sock

saw

sail

salt

sand

seal

safe

sink

WORKSHEET 3

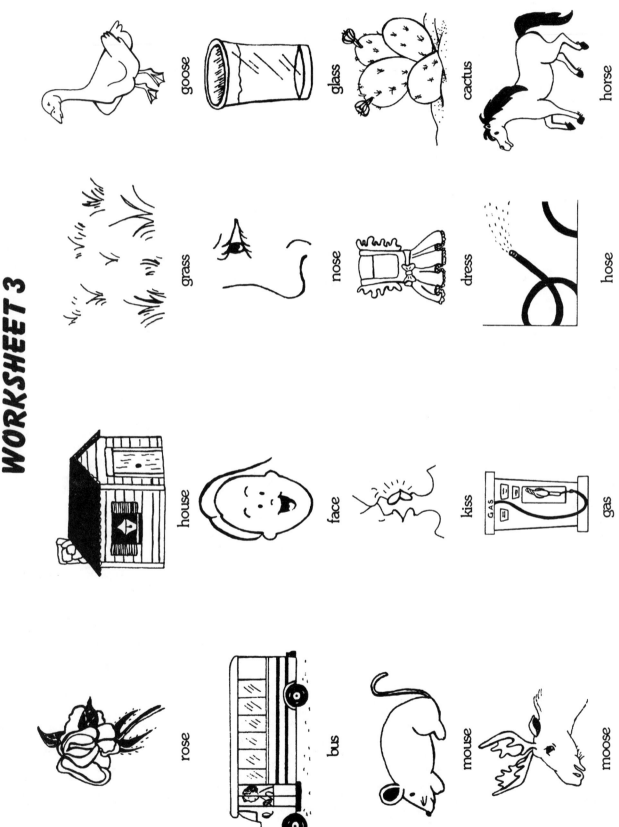

goose

glass

cactus

horse

grass

nose

dress

hose

house

face

kiss

gas

rose

bus

mouse

moose

WORKSHEET 4

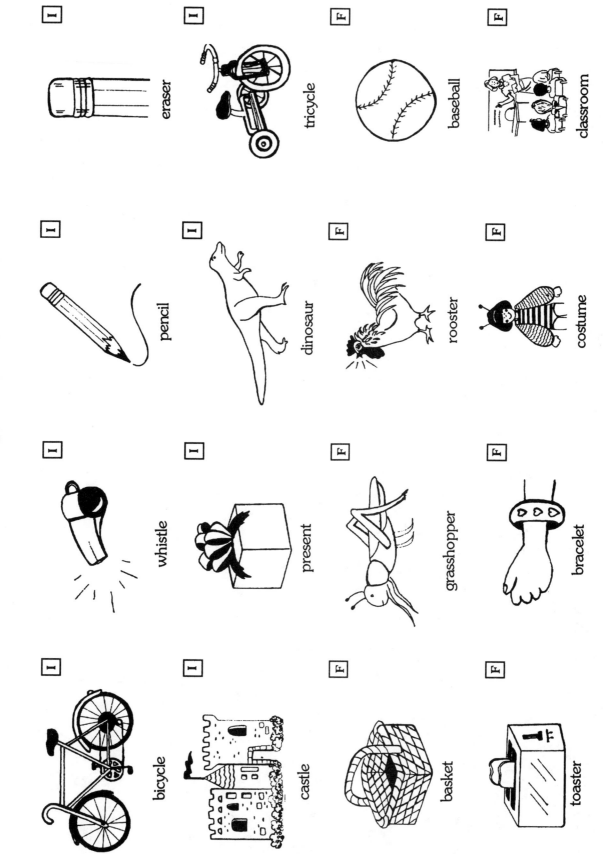

I eraser	I tricycle	F baseball	F classroom
I pencil	I dinosaur	F rooster	F costume
I whistle	I present	F grasshopper	F bracelet
I bicycle	I castle	F basket	F toaster

WORKSHEET 5

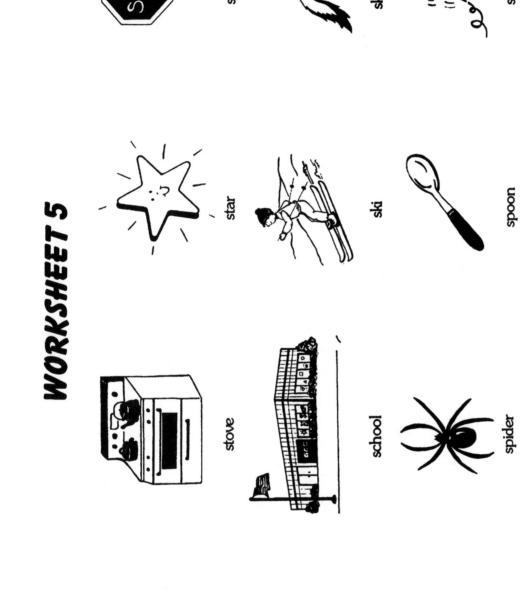

stop

skunk

spin

sweater

star

ski

spoon

swing

stove

school

spider

switch

step

skate

spill

sweat

WORKSHEET 6

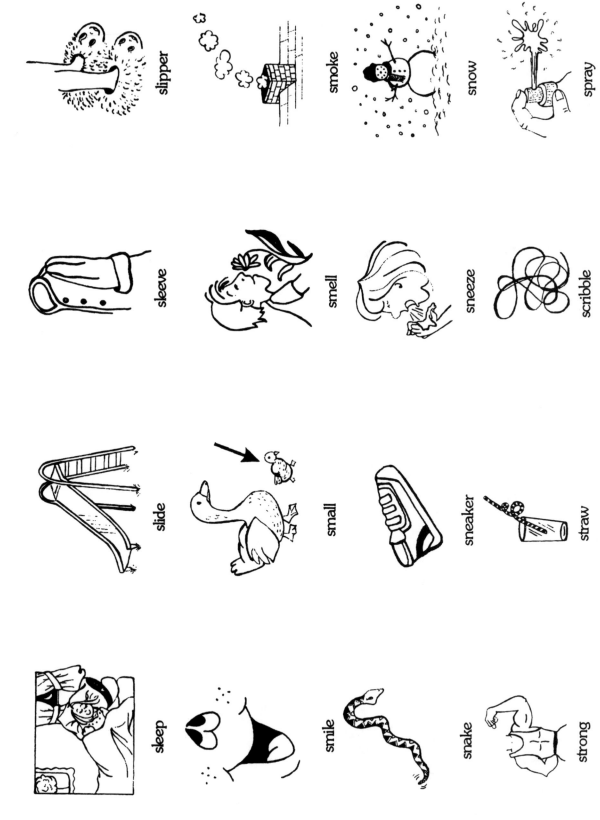

slipper

smoke

snow

spray

sleeve

smell

sneeze

scribble

slide

small

sneaker

straw

sleep

smile

snake

strong

WORKSHEET 7

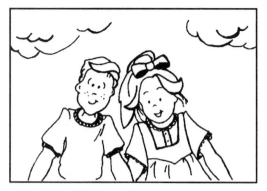

Susie likes to play with Sam.
Sam is Susie's best friend.

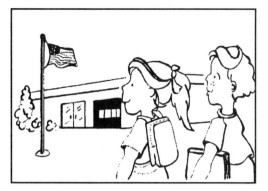

Susie and Sam are seven years old.
They go to the same school.

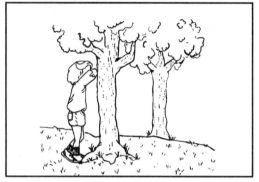

Sam's favorite game is hide-and-seek.

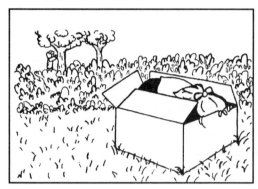

Sam closes his eyes.
Susie hides inside a box.

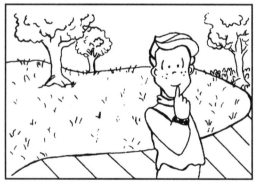

Sam counts to 10. He looks for Susie.

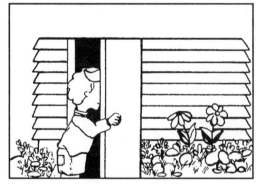

He searches in the house.
She is not inside.

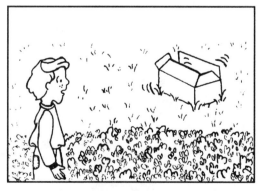

He searches outside.
Suddenly he sees the box move.

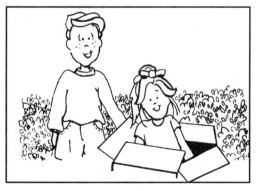

He runs to the box.
He smiles when he finds Susie.

81

WORKSHEET 8

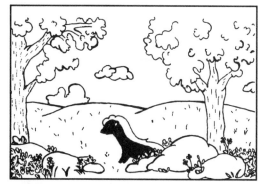

Smelly is a skunk. He is a smart skunk.

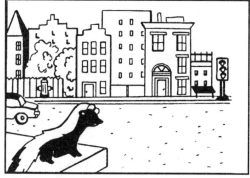

One day Smelly went to the city.
He wanted to visit the zoo.

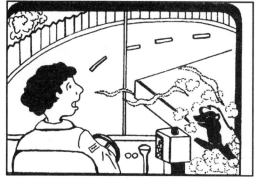

Smelly saw a bus. He got on the bus.

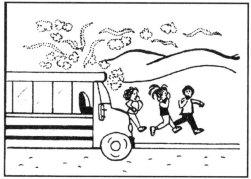

Everyone on the bus screamed.
They ran off the bus.

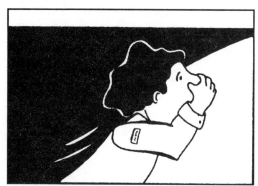

The bus driver ran off the bus.
He was holding his nose.

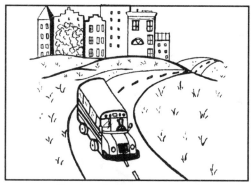

Smelly decided to drive the bus.
He drove safely.

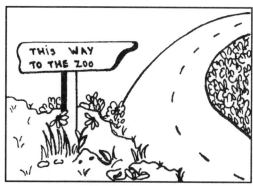

He saw a sign. It said, "This way
to the zoo."

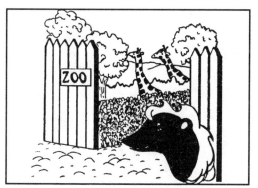

Smelly was the first skunk to ever drive
a bus to the zoo. He is very smart.

WORKSHEET 9

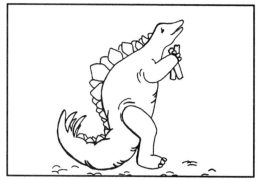

Sandy is a dinosaur. She bought two tickets for the circus.

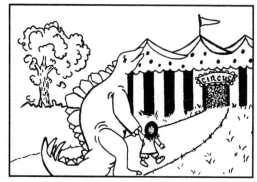

Sandy invited Sara to the circus. Sara wanted to go to the circus.

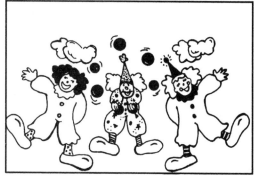

Sara wanted to see the clowns. So did Sandy.

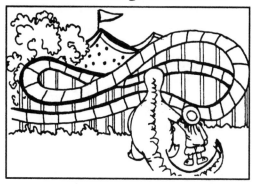

Sara wanted to try the roller coaster. Sandy was a little scared.

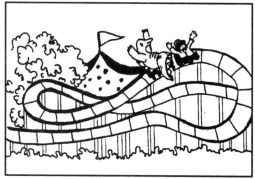

They sat in their seats. The roller coaster went up slowly.

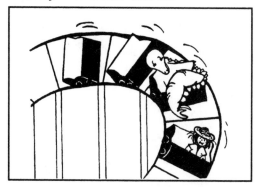

The roller coaster zoomed down fast.

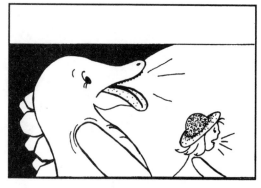

Sara and Sandy screamed. They were so scared.

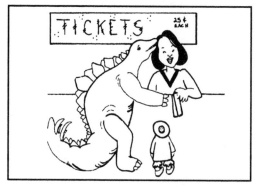

The roller coaster stopped. "That was awesome," said Sara and Sandy. Guess what? They decided to go on again!

APPENDIX B

GOAL

The child will learn to use sssss in conversation all the time.

MATERIALS

- 60 pennies
- 10 nickels
- Two clear cups. One cup should have a picture of a happy face drawn on it.
- Prize which the child will earn. The prize need not be expensive. The child should select the prize. Examples: a special doll or action figure, game, toy, a trip to the movies, clothing, etc.

LESSON TIME

Approximately one month

WHAT TO DO

Step One　Place the 60 pennies in the clear cup without the happy face. Place the 10 nickels next to the cup.

Show the nickels and the cup with the 60 pennies to the child. Tell the child he is going to try to win all the pennies that are in the cup. Tell him that he will win a penny each time he uses his good sssss when he talks. Each time he wins a penny he will put it into the happy face cup. After he wins all the pennies and nickels he will win a prize of his choice.

Ask the child what prize he would like to win. You might want to take a trip to a store so that he can show you what he wants. The prize should be something the child will be motivated to win. As you do Lesson 15, you will be frequently reminding the child what he is working to win. If the child has a picture of what he wants you can tape the picture on the second cup instead of drawing a happy face on it.

⇩　　⇩　　⇩　　⇩　　⇩

Step Two　It is very important that you monitor, or listen carefully to, the child whenever he is speaking. The sssss occurs frequently in English. The more often you catch and correct the child's errors, the faster he will learn to use sssss in conversation. As you start the penny program, realize that the child will lisp more often than he uses sssss. This is normal. He will gradually replace the lisp with sssss as you correct his errors and reinforce his use of sssss with praise and the earning of pennies. Once the child has earned all his pennies he will be ready for Step Three. If you find it too difficult to monitor the child throughout the entire day, you can start out by correcting or reinforcing correct use of sssss during specific periods, such as mealtimes, for the first couple of days. Increase your monitoring from mealtimes to an entire half day, for no more than two more days. Your next increase will be to monitor the child throughout as much of the day as possible.

If the child is in preschool or daycare for most of the day, speak to the person caring for the child. Tell this person that the child is learning to use his sssss sound in conversation. Give the caretaker a small notebook. Ask her to watch the child when he talks. Whenever she hears and sees him using his correct sssss, she should praise him and record his using sssss by drawing a star in the notebook for each time he used sssss. If the child used sssss five times, then the notebook should have five stars drawn in it. When you pick the child up, ask the caretaker how the child did using sssss during the day. Look at the small notebook with the child and count the number of stars the caretaker made. Praise the child for using sssss. When you get home, place a penny in the cup for each star earned during the day.

WHAT TO DO WHEN THE CHILD CORRECTLY USES SSSSS

As you begin Lesson 15 you will need to give the child a penny **each time** he correctly uses sssss, **on his own,** when talking. As he begins to use sssss more often on his own, you will start to give him pennies less frequently. In other words, as he gets better at using sssss, challenge him subtly by giving him a penny after a few words of correct sssss. As time goes on and he uses sssss more often, you will give him a penny only after he has spoken for a couple of hours without lisping. As you get down to the last 10 pennies, you should be giving him a penny for correct sssss no more than three times a day.
How do you know if you are giving too few or too many pennies a day? The following will help you gauge how well you are challenging the child with the penny program:

> Two to three weeks after starting the penny program, the child should have earned 30 to 40 pennies and should be using sssss, in conversation, about 50 percent of the time.

> Four to five weeks after starting the penny program the child should have earned all the pennies and should be using sssss, in conversation, over 80 percent of the time.

It is also very important to praise the child. You can praise the child by saying, "Very good! You remembered to say your sssss sound. You said, _____ (repeat sssss word your child said correctly)." The child will enjoy placing the penny in the cup by himself. He will also enjoy looking in the cup to see how many pennies he has; looking in the cup is a good way for the child to **see** how he is doing. You can also count the chips with him every now and then. He will be pleased to count how many pennies he has earned.

WHAT TO DO WHEN THE CHILD LISPS IN CONVERSATION

As you start the penny program, expect that the child will lisp more often than he will use his correct sssss. When you hear his lisp, say, "You forgot to use your sssss. Let's say _____ (name the word that was lisped) using a good sssss sound." Say the word and ask your child to repeat it correctly (do not give him a penny). Praise the child and say, "Remember to say your sssss when you talk so you can win pennies. You don't get pennies when you forget to say sssss."

WHAT TO DO IF THE CHILD PURPOSELY SAYS A SSSSS WORD AND WANTS A PENNY

The child will be eager to earn pennies. As a result he may approach you and say, out of the blue, a word he knows contains sssss. He may remind you to give him a chip for saying sssss. Praise him for saying a good sssss. You may give him a chip the first couple of times he does this. After the first couple of times, tell him that from now on he gets a penny only when he is talking, not for thinking of a sssss word to tell you.

WHAT TO DO IF THE CHILD ATTACHES SSSSS TO WORDS THAT DO NOT HAVE A SSSSS SOUND

Some children overgeneralize when learning when to use their sssss sound. In other words, they are not sure which words have a sssss sound so they use sssss randomly on all words. For example, a child might say "ssssbig." You can help the child get over this difficulty by doing the following:

1. Tell the child there is no sssss in *big*. Tell him we say *big*.
2. Ask the child to repeat the word correctly —*big*.

⇩   ⇩   ⇩   ⇩   ⇩

Step Three

This step is designed to help make the child more aware of those times he may still lisp. Once the child has earned all 60 pennies, he will be ready to earn nickels. Unlike pennies, which could only be won, nickels can be won or lost. In other words, when the child correctly uses sssss for a few hours, he earns a nickel and places it with the pennies in the happy face cup. However, if he lisps, he has to take the nickel out of the happy face cup and return it to the original cup.

Congratulate the child for working so hard and winning all his pennies. Tell him that he is almost ready to win his prize. Remove all the pennies from the happy face cup. Place 10 nickels in the empty penny cup. Show the nickels to the child and tell him that when all the nickels are in the happy face cup, he will get his prize. Tell him he wins a nickel for using his sssss just like when he won pennies. But if he forgets to use his sssss he has to take a nickel out of the happy face cup and put it back in the other cup. Show him how this works by saying and doing the following:

1. "Let's say you're talking and you use sssss a lot. You win a nickel." (Place a nickel in the happy face cup.)
2. "But let's say you're talking and you forget to use sssss and say 'thun' instead of 'sun.' If you say 'thun' I have to take one nickel out of the happy face cup and put it back with the other nickels.

(Take a nickel out of the happy face cup.) But if you remember to use your good sssss again, you can win back the nickel."

3. "Remember to use your sssss so that you don't have to lose any nickels."

4. Write down each sssss word the child incorrectly says. At the end of the day go over the list with the child. Say, "Today you forgot to use your sssss for the words I wrote on this paper. We need to practice these words so that tomorrow you will say them correctly and you will not lose a nickel." Then ask him to say each word correctly five times in a row.

It is normal for the child to lose and earn nickels over the course of a few days. Each time a nickel is lost ask the child to say the word correctly. Remind him to think about using his good sssss so he will not have to lose nickels.

The child should finish the nickels and the sssss once he uses sssss 100% of the time. Once the child has earned all ten nickels, return to the person who worked on this program with your child. She will want to check your child's progress and give him a certificate of achievement for completing the program. After he is given the certificate, he can have the reward he has worked hard to earn.

MAKING SURE THE CHILD CONTINUES TO USE THE SSSSS SOUND

Congratulations to you and the child for having successfully corrected his lisp! Before you put this manual away, however, I would like to leave you with a few suggestions and words of advice regarding the child's newly learned sound.

- First, over the next few days give the child frequent praise for using his good sssss sound. Be generous with praise.
- Second, be on guard for an occasional lisp. If the child slips and lisps, bring the error to his attention. Gently tell him that he forgot to use his sssss when he said _____. Ask him to repeat the word with his sssss sound.

If you notice a gradual increase in lisping, I suggest that you begin a motivational program to get the child back on track. For instance, tell him that each morning he will get five nickels in his happy face cup. Tell him he will lose a nickel each time he forgets to use his sssss sound. He must have at least one nickel left in his cup at the end of the day in order to get a reward (such as ice cream, candy, watch a favorite TV program, etc.). After a day or two of getting rewards, reduce the nickels in his happy face cup to three. By reducing the number of nickels you are requiring him to make fewer errors in order to win a reward at the end of the day. Within a few days the child should be back on track.

ACTIVITIES & MATERIALS

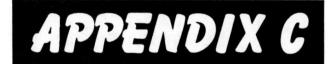

GAMES

Games are fun because they allow you and the child to play together by taking turns. Remember that taking a turn is used as a reward for success. For example, the child said sssss in isolation five times, as you asked him to do. He can take a turn. Then you take a turn. Taking a turn should also be a reward for effort even if the goal has not been met. Try to finish the lesson and the turn-taking activity at the same time. As you do the lessons there will be reminders to take turns at the turn-taking activity.

You can also make up your own board games. You will need a large piece of cardboard or poster board and markers or crayons. You draw a scene with a starting point and ending point. Draw a path divided into segments between the start and finish. Game pieces can be buttons, stones, or other small items. You can use dice or make a spinner. Homemade creative games are inexpensive and as much fun as store bought games.

The games listed below are appropriate for children ages four and older and can be found in most toy stores.

Boggle Junior
Bed Bugs
Ants in the Pants
Checkers
Crocodile Dentist
101 Dalmatians
Don't Wake Daddy
Hungry Hungry Hippos
Poppin' Magic
Squiggly Worms
Hi Ho! Cherry-O
Sound Safari
Oops & Downs
Goldilocks and the Three Bears Game
Don't Break the Ice
Animal Crackers Game
Snoopy's Doghouse Game
The Snoopy Game
How Does Your Garden Grow
Pick up sticks
Marbles

NONGAME ACTIVITIES

Nongame activities are completed by the child in segments. In other words the child does a portion of the activity as a reward for success. For example, if the child has selected Colorforms, he can place three or four colorform pieces on the background as a reward for saying sssss in isolation five times.

Colorforms
Magna Doodle
Etch A Sketch
Perler Beads
Luma Sketch
Tinkertoy
Lincoln Logs
Mr. Mighty Mind
Magna Shapes
Marble Works

CONVERSATIONAL MATERIALS AND ACTIVITIES

Conversational materials and activities are used to stimulate the child to talk. Engage the child in conversation as you play. Allow the child to take on whichever role he chooses (example: mechanic, doctor, dentist, etc.). The child should become involved in playing his part and conversing with you as you play your part. You can find many of the items for the activities around the house. Many can be found as children's play sets at most toy stores.

Play beauty parlor/barber shop
Play fix-it person
Play farm
Play garage mechanic
Play with Barbies, Ninja Turtles, Batman, etc.
Play restaurant
Play supermarket
Make believe cooking or baking
Have a tea party
Play birthday party
Play doctor or dentist office
Play secretary
Play police station
Play fire station
Play hospital
Play with the Playmobile figures and sets

LATERAL LISP SUPPLEMENT

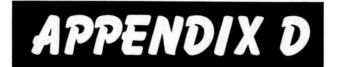

APPENDIX D

IDENTIFYING A LATERAL LISP

A lateral lisp occurs when air is emitted from the sides of the mouth, laterally, rather than frontally, through the front teeth. It is a sound that is hard to describe. It resembles a distorted "sh" sound. When producing a lateral lisp, the child lifts the middle of his tongue to the hard palate, thereby redirecting the forward flow of air out through the sides of his mouth. When correcting a lateral lisp, it is necessary to teach the child correct tongue position as well as how to direct the airflow frontally.

DIRECTIONS

It is recommended that this supplement be used by a speech pathologist. Once the lessons of this supplement have been completed the parent, an aide, or volunteer can take over and continue from Lesson Three of the manual. **Instruct the person taking over to read the Prelesson of the manual before working with the child.**

This supplement replaces Lessons One and Two of the manual which are designed to correct a frontal lisp. Once you have completed Lessons One and Two of this supplement return to the manual and begin Lesson Three. Lessons Three to Fifteen are appropriate for the correction of frontal and lateral lisps.

TONGUE, TEETH, AND LIP POSITIONING

 GOAL

You will teach the child to keep his teeth together, his tongue behind his teeth and his lips pursed.

 MATERIALS

Mirror
Worksheet 1
Marker or crayon

 LESSON TIME

10 minutes

WHAT TO DO

Sit next to the child. Place the mirror in front of you and the child. Look in the mirror, with the child, and say: "Look at my teeth. I'm going to make believe my teeth are doors. Look at my tongue. I'm going to make believe my tongue is a snake.

"When I open the doors (open teeth) you can see the snake (wiggle tongue). When the doors are open the snake is awake so he moves around (move tongue around inside mouth). Before I close the doors I make the snake lie down (place tongue at the bottom of mouth behind lower front teeth). Then I close the doors (place tongue at bottom of mouth and shut teeth with upper teeth overlapping lower teeth). When the doors are closed the snake cannot come out so he lies down (place tongue at bottom of mouth and shut teeth).

"Watch my mouth again. When I open the doors (open teeth slightly) the snake moves around (move tongue around inside mouth). When my teeth are closed the snake lies down (place tongue at bottom of mouth, behind lower front teeth, and shut teeth).

"Now it's your turn. Show me how you open your doors. Good job. Now show me how the snake can move around when the doors are open. Good. Now lay the snake down. Now shut the doors. Will the snake move around? No. Let's try opening the doors again but this time only a little bit. Show me how the snake can move around. Very good. Now lay the snake down and shut the doors. Will the snake move around? No.

"Did you know that snakes live in the ground? Look at my lips. I am going to make my lips look like a hole that a snake lives in in the ground (purse lips). Show me how you make a snake hole. Very good. Let's try making a snake hole again. Very good." If the child has difficulty pursing his lips see Troubleshooting.

"Show me again what the doors look like when they are closed. Is the snake lying down? Yes. Now keep the doors closed and make a snake hole. Good. The snake is lying down behind the closed doors in the snake hole.

"Let's practice making a snake hole while the doors are closed and the snake is lying down. Every time you make a snake hole with the doors closed we will color a happy face in one of the circles" (Worksheet 1, page 69 in manual).

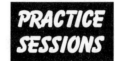

Repeat this lesson twice a day until you feel the child is ready to move on to
Lesson Two.

TROUBLESHOOTING

Some children have difficulty pursing their lips upon request. You
can help the child by doing the following:

1. Ask the child to "close the doors" (teeth closed with upper front
   teeth overlapping the lower front teeth).
2. Place a straw, cut to about three inches, against his closed front
   teeth. Ask the child to hold the straw with his lips.
3. Repeat 1 and 2 above a few times.
4. Ask the child to "make a snake hole" without the straw.

Return to the lesson once the child is able to purse his lips without
using the straw.

PRODUCING THE SSSSS SOUND

2

GOAL

You will teach the child how to
make the sssss sound.

MATERIALS

Turn-taking activity
Mirror

LESSON TIME

15 minutes

WHAT TO DO

Step One   Place the mirror in front of you and the child. Tell the child that you are going to make the snake sound. Tell the child to <u>listen carefully and watch you. Place your teeth together, purse your lips and make an sssss sound. Repeat a few times.</u>

Tell the child that you could make the snake sound because the snake was lying down, the doors were closed and your lips looked like a snake hole.

⇩   ⇩   ⇩   ⇩   ⇩

Step Two   Ask the child to look in the mirror. Then ask him to make the snake sound with you and to make his sssss so it sounds just like yours. Together make the sssss sound a few times. Allow the child to take a turn at the activity he selected. Then you take a turn. If the child lateralizes or is unclear, see Troubleshooting. If his sssss sounds good, continue to Step Three.

⇩   ⇩   ⇩   ⇩   ⇩

Step Three   Ask the child to make the snake sound alone. If he is successful ask him to make five sssss sounds in a row. Take turns at the activity. Continue this step until either the game is over or the child has lost interest.

If, on his own, the child reverts back to a lateral lisp, return to making the sound together. Make sure the child's lips are pursed. Take turns at the turn-taking activity. Repeat this step as often as necessary until the child is able to produce sssss on his own.

The child will need to practice producing sssss over the next two days before you move on to the next lesson. The idea is to carry over and reinforce correct production of the sssss sound.

Practice Session 1 is done the day after the lesson. Practice Session 2 is done the day after Practice Session 1. As much time should be spent on the Practice Sessions as was spent on the lesson. If you are unable to do the practice sessions with the child try to enlist another adult such as a parent, aide, or adult volunteer.

👍   👌   👍   👌   👍

**Practice
Session 1**

Repeat the lesson once in the morning and once in the afternoon.

👍   👌   👍   👌   👍

**Practice
Session 2**

You will need about 10 pennies.

Face the child so that he can see your mouth. Tell the child that you and he are going to play the "Catch Me" game. Tell him that you will try to trick him and he has to catch you. Tell the child that each time he catches you he will win a penny.

Tell the child that sometimes you will say sssss the right way (demonstrate). When you say sssss the right way he should say, "Good talking." If he catches you saying sssss the right way he will win a penny. Then tell him that sometimes you will say sssss the wrong way. Tell the child that instead of sssss you will say "sh" (demonstrate by making a lateral lisp). When you say a lateral lisp he has to catch you. When he catches you he says, "Wrong." Tell the child that he will win a penny when he catches you saying sssss the wrong way. When he catches you saying "sh" (lateral lisp) ask him to help you say it correctly. Then say sssss together. Do a couple of practice trials with the child, using pennies, so that you are sure he understands what he has to do when you say sssss and a lateral sssss. Switch roles after the child has caught you a few times. This time the child tries to trick you. The child will enjoy giving you pennies for catching him say sssss correctly and incorrectly. Play "Catch Me" for about ten minutes.

TROUBLESHOOTING

Some children do not make a clear sssss sound because either their tongue is not in the correct position or they do not direct the air flow frontally.

If the child's tongue position is incorrect do the following:

1. Place a small dab of jelly behind the child's lower front teeth.
2. Ask the child to touch the jelly with his tongue. The child's tongue should now be at the bottom of his mouth. Using the mirror, show the child where his tongue should be when he shuts his teeth.
3. Ask the child to shut his teeth. Remind him to keep his tongue down while touching the jelly spot when he says sssss.
4. Ask the child to "make a snake hole" (demonstrate by pursing your lips with the child) and make the sssss sound with you.

Repeat numbers 1-4, above, a few times. When you feel the child is ready, do only numbers 3 and 4, above. If he succeeds in making a clear sssss without the jelly, return to Step Two of the lesson. If his sssss still sounds lateralized or is not yet clear continue to do numbers 1-4 until he is able to produce a clear sssss without the jelly. Then return to Step Two of the lesson.

If the child's air flow is not directed frontally do the following:

1. Ask the child to "lay the snake down" (tongue should be down behind lower front teeth) and "close the doors" (upper front teeth should overlap the lower).
2. Ask the child to "make a snake hole" with you. As he purses his lips place a straw (cut to about three inches) in the opening of his mouth.
3. Ask the child to hold the straw with his lips.
4. Remind him to keep his tongue down and his teeth closed. Ask the child to make the snake sound come out of the straw as you and he say sssss together.

Repeat numbers 1-4, above, a few times. Then try number 4 above **without using the straw**. When he succeeds in making a clear sssss without the straw, return to Step Two of the lesson. If his sssss still sounds lateralized or is not yet clear, continue to do numbers 1-4 until he is able
to produce a clear sssss without the straw. Then return to Step Two of the lesson.

NOTES

NOTES

NOTES

NOTES

NOTES

NOTES

NOTES

NOTES